TIMELESS
WOMEN SPEAK

feeling
Youthful
at any
age

Nancy D. O'Reilly, PsyD • Margaret U. Castrey

Women Speak

Timeless Women Speak: Feeling Youthful at Any Age
By Nancy D. O'Reilly, PsyD & Margaret U. Castrey

Library of Congress Cataloguing-in-Publications Data
Library of Congress Control Number: 2008935805
Nancy D. O'Reilly, PsyD & Margaret U. Castrey
Timeless Women Speak: Feeling Youthful at Any Age
ISBN: 978-0-9820788-0-8
Library of Congress subject headings:
1. Health 2.Wellness
2008

Contents

Dedication

. . . .

I dedicate this book to Bee Payne Stewart, to my three daughters, Lauren, Leigh, and Ragan, and to all the other wonderful women who dared to speak of their concerns and fears as well as their joys and blessings. Together, we will help one another live fuller and happier lives. I also dedicate this book to my granddaughters, Alexis, Isabel, Patty June, Dain, and soon-to-arrive baby Sky in the hope that they will continue the important work of empowering women.

Acknowledgments

It is hard to believe that it has been almost 10 years since I began the research for the WomenSpeak Project. I started from my own personal need and ended up doing it for all the women I came to know during my research. I acknowledge my tremendous gratitude to and appreciation of the thousand women who were directly surveyed and the hundreds of women from our focus groups and the Web site who took the time to participate in our study to share their hearts and fears with us. They answered the hard questions about their own aging process and how they really felt about aging in a society that pooh-poohs getting older.

I want to thank all the women in my life, especially my sister Steff who never stopped believing in me. I want to thank my mother, Phyllis, who looks me in the eye and tells the truth. I want to thank my daughters, Lauren, Leigh, and Ragan, who encouraged me and inspired me to keep going and shared so very much of themselves. I want to thank my good friends, Mary Beth, Linda, all my Nancy friends, and Agnes, my sweet Canadian friend who always makes me smile and never let me give up.

Thanks to my co-author and editor, Maggie. You are the best of all things that has happened to me during this time. You helped me focus and you made me look good. You brought to the research and book your heart and with it, a deep, committed passion for this work. You are truly my good friend and you exude what I think all women should aspire to be: kind, generous, creative, warm, intelligent, and unselfish. You let me take the limelight and I know you were the "wind beneath my wings." I am so grateful you came into my life.

I also want to thank Burrell Behavioral Health for the help of their staff and a very special psychologist and administrator who assisted us with all the research and design. Paul Tomlinson, PhD., is one of the many professionals who help us to better understand our world. As Paul said so many years ago, "You have to eat an elephant one chunk at a time." Well, we did just that.

I want to thank Larry, the man I have been married to for 39 years. We have literally grown up together and had to do some real work to get it done. I thank you for your support and love, and for sharing the covers and letting me put my cold feet on you to get warm on a cold winter night. You supported, you pushed, you challenged me, and helped me to believe in myself at times when I was tired and down. Larry never quits and he taught me to never give up; the prize is too important and the end can and does have sweet rewards.

Last but not least, thank you, little girls, the next generation of women who will make this world a better place: my granddaughters, Alexis, Isabel, Patty June, Dain, and soon-to-arrive baby Sky. You all bring a special kind of inspiration to me. I understand now why God gave me daughters and granddaughters. We have much work to do for all women.

Introduction

I am a lucky woman. I can hide from winter in a home by the ocean and set time aside to write, to paint, and to think about my life and my purpose. Each of us must find her own purpose; my challenge is to slow down and try not to be in such a hurry to read the next chapter of my life.

Such interesting chapters have unfolded already. I never thought I would have three beautiful daughters, that I would have four, soon to be five, precious granddaughters, or that I would become a fierce and dedicated advocate for women. I have learned never to use the word "never." I now use the written word and even advocate politically for women's rights and to improve our quality of life. I believe in women and that each one of us deserves to be happy, healthy, and have bundles of self-esteem. I have focused my career, beliefs, and convictions — and all my energy and time training and educating myself — on this book and this path that I have chosen to follow. I am also banking my reputation and my career on one task and passion: to share with this world the importance and uniqueness of women. Yes, I am all about empowering and elevating women to the level of respect and admiration they deserve.

More than 10 years ago, I started to face the issues and concerns about growing older that were increasingly affecting my life. I began this journey when I was about to turn 50; now I am about to turn 60. Where has the time gone?

In my youth, I never allowed age to affect me and was sure I could easily ace the aging process. I believed women who were aging badly were just not trying hard enough. Surely if they had my discipline and determination they would have stayed youthful and vibrant. Today as I look back I can honestly say I have had to eat my words. I take back what I have said and hope everyone to whom I expressed this view will forgive me. I apologize: Was I ever wrong! I have learned that women speak the truth when they say, as Bette Davis did: "Old age is no place for sissies." I was not at all prepared to lose my youthful bloom; no one I truly trusted had ever told me the truth about this uncharted territory.

I found myself feeling nervous and alone with my deflated ego. I felt embarrassed, as if I had discovered spinach between my teeth after I had been grinning and talking loudly, certain that I was impressing everyone in the room with my foolproof plan to beat aging. In my discovery process, I found aging was not nearly as easy as it sounds. Until we get there, most of us can't understand it or really relate to the experience. Recently my 88-year-old mother told me: "All things are relative to where you are in life." I never believed her when I was younger but now I am a believer. Thanks, Mom. You were right. Mom also told me recently, "You know, Nancy, I did not mean to get old, it just happened." I will never forget those words because now I know what she means.

Having discovered that I can't avoid getting older, I want to learn to live in the here and now. I need to know I am present and available to my experiences. And I want to believe I have made a difference for others.

MY STORY

I arrived in this world as a hairless, scrawny, less-than-cute three-pound premature baby girl. There were no pictures of me until I was six months old, which no doubt proves how non-photogenic I was. My parents were told premature babies usually did not survive and to be prepared for my possible demise. They did not worry for long because they quickly noticed my large mouth, healthy lungs, and well-developed vocal cords. Each time they visited my incubator they found me kicking my legs and making loud noises. Since that beginning I have continued to use my verbal and physical attributes to pursue my goals.

This energy and enthusiasm has helped me and probably also hurt me. I enjoyed carrying a big stick and raising eyebrows with my (sometimes politically incorrect) declarations. As a child I was a total tomboy, meaning I did not behave in ways that were gender-specific. I ignored my wise grandmother when she would ask me, "Did you show your petticoat, Nancy?" I was told that the *normal* girls wanted to play with dolls, stay clean, and learn important life skills like cooking and sewing, all of which bored me to death and sounded like far too much hard work. I found other things much more exciting: playing kickball and baseball, building forts, digging and crawling into caves. The neighbor boys knocked on my door all the time asking me to come out and play. Life was great! I really didn't know I was different from the boys until I was nine and my friend Jimmy asked if I could spend the night at his house. When I asked my mother she looked stunned and shocked by my request. What could be wrong? What had I said that caused such a reaction? Since I knew my mother was perfect and so very wise, I assumed there must be something wrong with me. Thus began my gradual realization that girls are different from boys.

As a girl soon to be woman, I needed to find out how to fit into this foreign female world. My older sister Stephany shared my mother's sentiments and said to me one day: "Nancy, when are you ever going to be a girl?" Boy, that was a real shocker. I thought she was a perfectly prissy girl so she must know what she was talking about. I had a strange feeling I was in for trouble, but since I could still kick a ball farther than the boys on my block, surely growing up would be a piece of cake … wouldn't it?

Girl territory held no appeal for me because I perceived our society did not really value girls. I remember listening to people talking about how much they hoped their next child would be a boy and that life with a Bob or Joe Junior would be so grand. I did not hear anyone say, "Oh my, how exciting, she had a girl!" I think my basic understanding came from the difference I was told existed between the two sexes — that boys were rough and tumble and girls were sweet and looked pretty. Of course, I had heard about "Sugar and spice and everything nice" and that women needed to be quiet, reserved, pleasant, and attractive. This was clearly not me. I felt so odd in my female skin. I was sure every other girl was doing a much better job being female than I was. I think that's when I became interested in learning why I felt that way. I have continued to do that every day of my life.

As I grew up, I tried to prepare myself for the inevitable. If I had to be a girl I needed to figure out how to stand out from all the rest, both men and women. I was a competitive young woman, although I am not sure that got me a lot of points. Women were not supposed to be overtly competitive. It was, as I was told, *not ladylike*. Gads, what did *that* mean? I really liked men's honest, open, and frank way of just getting in each other's faces and saying, "I'm going to beat your a--," while smiling at the same time. I thought that was a cool and upfront way to handle things.

I was fine with not getting invited to a lot of girl parties (OK, so it did hurt my feelings a little to be excluded). But most of my friends growing up were male, fun, and direct, and I liked that until they started acting funny. What in the world had happened to my guy friends? They had become silly, had trouble talking to me, and would no longer look me in the eye. What had I done to deserve this behavior?

Soon I found they did not want to hang out anymore but wanted to go on a *date*. The rules changed quickly after that and now I not only felt strange in my female skin, but much worse, the guys I had so enjoyed before had become babbling idiots. The fun had ended; a new game and era had begun, and I was really not having any fun at all, so I channeled my energies into working out. In the course of changing from a tomboy into a teenaged girl, I had somehow internalized society's messages about the importance of a woman's appearance.

As a workout queen, I religiously went to the gym each day, knowing and praying that with each two-hour workout of aerobics, running, and weight training I would emerge fit and beautiful…a shining example of a woman. This was my way of ensuring that I was — and would always be — engaging and attractive for eternity. I assumed the planning and hard work that I invested in staying young and beautiful meant those traits would always be mine.

My twenties were a blur. I went from sorority life and the college dorm to marriage with Larry just a few months before my twenty-first birthday. My first child was on the way. I had a college degree in my sights and now I was having a baby. I had no idea how this would affect my life. I was basically clueless and, as you may recall, I had no domestic skills. I began practicing my cooking skills on my dad that summer and assumed I was making progress because I did not kill him, which gave me hope.

I had goals and objectives and remained determined that marriage and a baby would not deter me from reaching them. I had a lot to learn in a very short period of time. I had been an independent woman and being married and pregnant with no money was not to my liking. I began a part-time job to bring in some cash even though my energy was dwindling as my pregnancy progressed. Lauren arrived and parenting began. Larry and I brought her home and the first thing we did was almost drown her. We both failed to notice we had not screwed the cap on her bottle. Poor Lauren was our experiment in parenting. We have apologized to her many times for our ignorance. The good news is, she survived and is thriving in

Los Angeles. Her sister Leigh was born two years later and Ragan was born four years after that. We had a house full of girls and Larry was thinking "girl's basketball team." He ended up being a great coach for them.

During this time, I was making my way, juggling my many roles and jobs as mother, student, and wife. Having girls challenges a mother to think about the female world and what kind of life they will have, and I studied hard to earn a university degree for each daughter. When I was working on my doctorate, people asked, "Why do you work so hard?" "How can you justify taking so much time and energy away from your children, husband, cats, dogs, and community service?" And my personal favorite, "Why aren't you at home?" I have no regrets and would do it all again for one simple and important reason. I had a profound need to show women we could do it all if we just kept pursuing and achieving our dreams and goals. I wanted — thought other women wanted and *needed* — positive female role models and mentors to show them the way.

I wanted to set an example for my girls that they could do anything and I hoped my education and my career would be a testament to what was possible: that they could accomplish any dream. To this day, I want my girls, granddaughters, and all women to know that. This book is for them and all women who want to have a voice and a sense of their own worth.

Speaking of self-worth, while studying to become a psychologist, I learned about Freud's view that having been born without a penis makes women insecure and less than men. When a psychology professor told me I had *penis envy*, I retorted, "Why would I have penis envy when I can have all the penises I want?" Unfortunately, his displeasure with my remark showed up in my final grade.

I began my twenties as an independent free thinker, who thought she knew it all. I ended my twenties less confident, more thoughtful, and knowing that each year would bring many life lessons. I learned a lot about humility. I had to learn to live with someone, share, be cooperative, be considerate of others' feelings, and not have to be right all the time.

My thirties are a little clearer to me than my twenties. On my thirtieth birthday my girls were 10, 8, and 4 years old. I had it made. They were doing well and I was working as a therapist and felt good about my appearance. I was confident about my accomplishments. I had completed my master's in guidance and counseling. I was on my path to make the world a better place and decided I needed to get the ultimate degree. I began working on my doctorate, a journey I will never forget. It changed my entire view of people and the world. I had always believed I was open-minded and that there was goodness in all people. I knew I could help *anyone* if I just tried hard enough. I had a huge education ahead of me.

My husband was busy building the family business. Our girls were busy with school and activities 24/7: tennis, track and field, basketball, and so on. With no free nights and little time for ourselves much less a date night, our marriage suffered. Larry and I continued to parent while realizing we would have to grow up in this relationship because we both were so young and ill prepared for marriage and childrearing. We learned; we fought; we separated. Our separation ended up being a good thing. Each of us found ourselves and then we went looking for each other. The old saying, "If you let something go and it comes back to you, it will be yours forever" seems to be true for us. Our marriage grew stronger and we were becoming friends who did not take each other for granted. At that time I truly felt complete; I looked good, felt capable, and I was full of hope for my future.

My forties opened my eyes. After my husband went through a tough midlife crisis at age 40, I assumed I would head down the same path. I did not like the sound of it or the implications. I was determined to stop the clock and fight the signs of aging. I remember thinking "I will be different from other women. I will not let age affect me." I worked out a couple of hours each day. I haunted cosmetic counters in search of magical products. I worked on the flab and still the extra pounds came. I tried running and hit the aerobics floor sweating to the tune of "YMCA." I was determined I would be admired and no one would ignore me when I entered a room. But I was in my early forties with teenaged kids. It really changed my world to see my daughters exemplify the youthful bloom I was losing. All of my girls were gorgeous athletes and physically fit. I was so jealous of their beautiful, youthful bodies. Was I as attractive as they? Was I less interesting? What was going on with me? I feared losing control of my life and especially my youthful looks. I remember walking into a room with my girls and feeling all eyes on them and none on me. I felt I had been dismissed. I had begun to feel invisible to others. Was I the only one experiencing this? I was definitely *not* prepared to feel like the disappearing woman.

That was when I began to wonder what in the world was wrong with me. I had spent my life helping men and women with their self-esteem. I worked with them to overcome all their negative self-talk and work on their self-images. I had taught them strategies to identify their "Stinken Thinken" and to use positive self-statements to feel better about themselves. Now I had the same problem. Why was I having trouble? I wondered if other women were feeling this way. It did not help even when Larry assured me I was pretty and still sexy. Our lives were full and he was still going strong with the family business. I was finishing my doctorate, working, and watching my life fly by.

I was almost 50 years old when I decided to leave my position as the director of the employee assistance program of a large healthcare system. I was responsible for over 100,000 lives. We were understaffed and I had to balance my work as a half-time psychologist and a half-time administrator. I was finding it really hard to juggle all of those balls and I was starting to drop some. Sometimes dropping a ball is a good way to re-focus and re-evaluate a next move.

The biggest ball dropped when my oldest daughter Lauren was in a serious car accident and I took a leave of absence to care for her. Thank God, she survived her injuries and made what was said to have been a remarkable recovery. I was thrilled and felt blessed.

Then it was back to *my* issues: I just couldn't make myself go back to work. It was time to make a change. Lauren's accident had clearly created a time for me to refocus my life, which allowed me to think about what was really important. (I realized later I was having that much-dreaded midlife crisis.)

On my fiftieth birthday I actually ran away to our home on the ocean. I had decided I would not risk the chance Larry might have a surprise party for me. I had surprised him on his fortieth and his fiftieth birthdays and I assumed it was payback time. I spent my fiftieth birthday alone, feeling sorry for myself and feeling depressed and confused. Not a very healthy or pretty picture for a clinical psychologist.

As I sat by the sea, I admitted to myself that I was really scared about losing my identity as a psychologist. I wondered what it would be like to not have a job to go to: "Could I just be Nancy, whoever she was?" I knew I would find something; I made a pact with myself to wait and not be in too big a hurry about what I would do next.

When I was working on my third degree (a doctorate in clinical psychology) one of my professors told our class, "Whatever you decide to do with your education, *make a contribution!*" That statement hit me hard. I decided this would be my mantra, and that concept drives my actions and pursuits to this day.

During all the time my self-esteem was becoming vested in my life as a psychologist, it continued to be closely intertwined with my appearance. I began to realize the clock was working against me, just as it did for everyone else. Looking at my image in the mirror made me wonder: Who is that person? Do I even like her? I began to avoid mirrors, especially if it meant standing next to a younger, beautiful woman applying makeup to her youthful face or brushing her long, shiny locks.

Why was I like this? My mother hated aging and getting older. She had celebrated more un-birthdays than I could count. She was never happy with growing older and never let anyone know her age. I knew my mother was 25 when she had my sister, which was the only clue I ever had to her age. Today my mother is 88 years old and she still does not celebrate her birthday.

My view of aging has a lot to do with my exposure to my mother's anti-aging view. My grandmother, Big Nancy, was a most positive female role model. She was a small woman who could command attention when she entered a room. She wanted the best table in the restaurant and that is where we went. I loved her style; she was a cool granny.

As a psychologist I knew I had to learn more, both for my own sake and for the sake of other women, including my daughters and granddaughters. I felt it was my duty to prepare them for what their lives would offer and warn them how our youth-oriented society rewards fresh beauty and punishes seasoned age. I felt one of my jobs as a woman and a professional was to grow personally, and then to share what I learned to help other women with the journey each one would take as she entered her middle years and beyond. That was a place foreign, unfriendly, and very much misunderstood. I hated to think I must tell a woman that all her years and experience were not necessarily going to be valued or appreciated. Many women I have spoken with feel guilty and ashamed that age has changed their youthful appearance and robbed them of their earlier energy and drive.

This issue was clearly larger than my own personal experience, so I decided to examine the feelings and thoughts of women of all ages to find out how they were handling aging issues in our society. Although no other woman had ever talked with me about this, I could not believe I was the only one afraid of feeling invisible and suffering from other consequences of aging.

I decided I would use my education and clinical experience to lead me to the resources I needed to find my answers. My quest for knowledge began with a visit to my local bookstores, and continued as I surfed the Web. I was looking for a book, a guide, anything that would tell me how others — women who were handling aging much better than I — had successfully entered into their middle years. Sadly, I found little that spoke to me or calmed my fears. Most of the books I found insulted my intelligence and left me with a bitter taste in my mouth. Some books said upfront that a woman had to avoid getting older at all costs, through the use of hormones, cosmetic procedures, and magical elixirs. Many books talked about ways to beat the clock, to hide the years or — if all else failed — told us to lie. These books reinforced the idea that their readers must stay young and beautiful if they wanted to be loved and that losing their youth and beauty would render them invisible. These books also implied that if you lost youth it was your own fault for not doing enough to avoid this terrible condition.

Many of these books were cute, flip, naïve, or too off-the-wall for me. I read about women's cults, becoming a goddess, and stories of crones that had lost their once-great, mystical powers and were now defined by men and fearful women as witches. I did not understand how any of this was going to help me and other women find some place to feel good about ourselves as we grew older. It really looked pretty bleak out there: we could either jump on the service-and-product train to arrive at the promised land, young, renewed and beautiful, assured of our continuing place in society, or we could shrink away into irrelevance.

I was getting more confused and angry that no one had taken the time to help women with these issues. I was sad and worried about my own future but more important, I feared for all women and their futures. Why was this important topic being ignored? Why hadn't researchers and educators conducted research that would help women prepare for the changes they would experience as they grew older? Surely, women of all ages needed to know and have their concerns and needs met. I had already discovered that there was little research about women's views of their own aging process. No one, including myself, knew how women really felt about their own aging process at 40, 50, 70, or even 80. I felt I had been given a job to do and this gave me a renewed sense of purpose. I decided to find out what women really thought. I wanted to know the truth: How do women feel about themselves as they age and what are the ingredients each one needs in order to age successfully? To me, that meant continuing to *feel* youthful regardless of my chronological age.

At last I knew how I would make my contribution. I would develop a survey to learn about women's perceptions of their own aging process. I called my project WomenSpeak because my purpose and mission was to get women of all ages to speak about their views and concerns about growing older.

THE RESEARCH

My research began when I started asking women ranging in age from 18 to 88 about their feelings, their perceptions, and their concerns about growing older in our society. I had already admitted it to myself: I was afraid of aging. To be completely honest, I needed to reassure myself I was not alone and losing my mind. My happy discovery was that most of the women I approached to participate in the research were at first surprised and then extremely pleased to have an opportunity to discuss their fears. So many women said, "I'm so glad you asked," or "I have never been asked anything like that," and always: "Thanks for asking." Women of all shapes, sizes, careers, and socioeconomic and educational backgrounds were eager to be a part of the WomenSpeak Project.

I spoke at many women's functions and meetings, and posted the survey on the newly formed Womenspeak.com Web site. The number of completed surveys grew to more than 1,000 (and by the way, women of all ages are still participating in this research).

The surveys confirmed I was not alone in my worries. Women of all ages said they were afraid of growing older in our youth-oriented society. In fact, nearly half of the women said they were actually afraid of getting older. That's half of all women we surveyed, including women in their twenties and wise and experienced women who had nearly completed long lives. The fear of aging cuts across all lines of age, education, marital state, sophistication, and even health status.

My fifties in many ways have been great and awful all at the same time. Learning to deal with my fears was, well, frightening! My experiences of talking and sharing with other women have made all the difference in helping me regain my self-esteem. Now, I have my voice… I am confident, I paint, I have passion, and I get to do what I want. My kids are great and my granddaughters are wonderful. I have a lot of women encouraging me to keep going and get this book written as I promised I would.

Although I am still in my fifties I am peering over the horizon at my sixtieth birthday. I am getting ready. I am working with a personal trainer to build up strength and have shed 16 pounds and returned to a healthy weight. Who knows, I may just throw *myself* a birthday party because after this book comes out, lying about my age will be an impossibility. But you know, 60 is looking pretty good and I think I will be pleased with the outcome.

THIS BOOK

I began working with my co-author, Margaret Castrey, when it was time to write up my research for a professional audience. We have continued to work together ever since, and she helped with the focus groups and the creation of this book.

This book is for all of these women. If you have ever wondered if you are the only woman struggling with getting older, this book is for you. If you plan on living past the age of 30 and are concerned about the emotional, psychological, and physical impacts of aging, read on. If you want to know what women honestly think about aging, they tell the truth in these pages. Most of all, read this book if you want the best for a daughter or granddaughter.

Let's not become invisible. Let's keep roaring about the power and wonder of women. We need each other to make a difference. Together we can express our fears and then chase them away. We are not anti-youth, we are pro-age! We want women to live their lives without fear and to have the resources and support they deserve whatever their age. Keep reading to hear how other women have learned to feel youthful at any age. You too can feel good about all the wisdom, skills, and talent you have acquired by living each day to the fullest.

Let us create a new heritage for the women of today and for the generations to come. I truly believe that knowledge bestows power. Women are the world's purchasing agents. We control over 85 percent of the economy's growth through the things we buy, service providers we employ, what we eat, where we sleep, and how we dress. We make most of the decisions about consumer products, and most of the major healthcare choices for our loved ones. Let's use this power to make sure woman are informed about their options, cared for, and encouraged about their long, healthy futures. We want women to be able to live, laugh, and love longer in lives full of passion and purpose. We want them to avoid feelings of fear or guilt when they no longer look youthful and vibrant. We want women to revel in their rich lives and treasure the experiences they have acquired on the way to becoming interesting and strong at every age.

This book seeks to fulfill that need with the stories of so many women who spoke openly about their concerns and fears of aging. I hope this book helps you find your voice so that you will become a mentor and guide for younger women. These women want and need you. They are standing behind you waiting to take up the baton for women and, in their turn, empower those behind them. But they need your help. After you read this book, please take the time to share your views and offer your voice on the Womenspeak.com Web site.

We know that women's hands do indeed rock the cradle. Let's reach out to each other and rock women's worlds!

AUGUST 2008

SPRINGFIELD, MISSOURI

CHAPTER 1 *Getting the Message:*
Stay Young
and Beautiful

Our society sells "youth" to us daily on the streets, on newsstands, on the radio, on our television screens, and even in casual conversations. Listen carefully to hear a quiet inner voice even now that says, "Stay young and beautiful if you want to be loved." A song on that subject was written in 1933, and the message is even more pervasive in our culture today. Many women in our society have adopted this as their theme song. They fear that by aging they will lose it all, and they feel ever more anxious because they do not know exactly what "it" is.

Women tell us they feel guilty without knowing why. Many of us are scared of being perceived as old. We are embarrassed and conceal what's happening to us, and then we judge ourselves and one another harshly. We second-guess ourselves: "Maybe I have not done enough, or tried hard enough, or prayed enough to stay young and beautiful." We feel guilty about our age and then feel guilty about feeling guilty. It's a classic no-win situation.

The crucial question for all women who are getting older (please note: this is all living women) is: What is left for women if they have tried everything? What if they have bought all the products, gone under the knife, swallowed all the youth-producing elixirs, pounded the gym floor, and cycled until our buns of steel cramped — and we still look and feel older?

Are we destined to become laughable, like the greeting cards that show aging women in ridiculous costumes? Are we left only with sadness, like the pitiful older women in pharmaceutical ads? Absolutely not!

WHAT THIS BOOK CAN DO

Women do not have to suffer alone, and this book intends to provide support and encouragement. It will show that many others share the same fears and concerns about growing older in a society that takes a dim view of aging. It is a guide to the changes women experience through each decade of life, told in women's own stories. It can help women overcome their isolation and feel connected to each other.

We invite women to start with the chapter for the age they are now, read the decade they will graduate into, and read about their daughters and mothers. For those who want more depth and detail, there's information about the WomenSpeak research and history of women. This is not intended to become a chore. Instead, we hope it will be a resource that helps women to feel good about their lives. By reading how other women handle their fears, relationships, health, and finances, women can imagine and create for themselves confident, fulfilled, and happy lives.

This is important. Women do not need to feel guilty about losing that youthful bloom, and we do not need to feel that we have failed when gravity exerts its inevitable influence on our bodies. This is a natural process that eventually happens to all of us, especially as each generation lives a little bit longer than the one before it.

Women can and do have wonderful lives as we get older and we can teach each other how to enjoy and glory in every year of our lives. This book — and the years of research that support it — came about because women don't talk honestly with each other about aging. Because we are embarrassed, many women won't talk about their personal aging concerns at all. We have been trained to believe that revealing our messy interior landscape is poor manners, so we have kept our fears locked away.

As researchers, we have found that when women are given the chance to talk about how they feel — with people who truly believe their thoughts and concerns matter — they open up. When women truly feel safe and let down their hair to tell their truths, they get *really* serious — and very verbal. In fact, once they start talking they have trouble stopping.

Women told us they are surprised and thrilled to be asked to talk about their fears and concerns about growing older. They tell us they want their lives to be different. We know from the candid women who took part in our research that about half of women of all ages are fearful and feel unprepared to meet the challenges of growing older. We also found the other half doesn't seem to have much trouble and takes it in stride.

This gave us the idea for this book. Women of every age who struggle with getting older need help. Why don't we team up and share the secrets of success so we can all age successfully and feel youthful at any age? Most of our mothers gave us little guidance about aging beyond telling us to accept it or ignore it.

. . . .

Why don't we team up to share and learn each other's secrets so we can all age successfully and feel youthful at any age?

. . . .

Today, in an entrenched beauty culture that worships the appearance of youth, women need to talk about the realities of aging and learn from each other how to cope. We all deserve lives that are rich in experience and feelings of satisfaction. By telling our truths we can add quality years to our lives. That's what this book intends to do.

THE VELVET ANCHOR HOLDS US DOWN

Recently I spoke to a group of young women preparing for their master's and doctoral degrees in clinical psychology. I was surprised to hear they did not feel supported by their female professors. They yearned for female mentors and someone to show them the way. They said the problem for women today is less the glass ceiling of the 1970s than what they called the "Velvet Anchor." These women said, "The problem is not so much the ceiling above us; what's worse is all the things that hold us down."

The Velvet Anchor is all the soft, silken, subtle, and in many cases subconscious, ideas we believe about what it means to be a woman. Today these ideas hold us down as much — or more — than the world around us.

Although it's surely true some men and some institutions block women's progress, what is more interesting to us are the ways in which women sabotage themselves and each other. Women need to understand the ways they hold themselves back and keep their daughters, their sisters, and all other women down. Women should not underestimate their ability to influence others: we can encourage and support or we can undermine and block other women's success.

It is up to all women to continue the pursuit of happiness and freedoms for women in this century. We live in a modern world but, until all women feel they have personal power to live and be what they choose, we are not finished. Women have the role and opportunity to teach the world about values and beliefs that will sustain and offer quality lives to all people.

I have worked with women of all ages for more than 25 years. I have watched women, including myself, do more and more all the time and add — never subtract — jobs from our lives. We seem to believe we need to do it all, which naturally causes us to worry about everyone and everything. Women are professional worriers who have cornered the market when it comes to worrying. Anyone who is tired of worrying can just ask another woman to take over. She is the expert and will know what to do.

In the course of my clinical practice and this research, I learned women worry about everyone except themselves. They worry about other people's health, happiness, and well-being, and they put a lot of energy into making things better for everyone else. When they do pay attention to themselves they go to the dark side: they worry about being alone, not being able to care for themselves, getting behind on their bills, and losing their youthful bloom.

One of the worst things about this kind of worrying is that it is so often fruitless. For a variety of reasons, women may feel unable to devise solutions to problems about which they feel fearful and emotional. This book seeks to address that and offer some solutions.

WHY WE ARE THE WAY WE ARE

If we are to get women feeling better about themselves, we need to understand where we have come from. In ancient times women customarily rested and hung out together when they were about to give birth or when they were menstruating. When in the menstrual tent, they were excused from housework and taking care of the family. This was a joyous time, free from the hard work of beating dirty clothes on the rocks or feeding the camels and the menfolk. This tradition worked well for ovulating and pregnant women and they were glad.

However, when a woman stopped ovulating she lost the right to enjoy the safety and security of the menstrual tent. Menopausal women were doomed in their later years to unceasing labor caring for the tribe. These once-proud and happy women were banished from the tent's safety and companionship and left with their memories and sadness at losing their honored place in society. This shows that our burdens of regret for getting old are very deep-seated.

Women historically have been dismissed for being female unless, like Helen of Troy, they are immortalized for their beauty. We are criticized for our hormones and condemned for our erratic emotions. The most enraging question a man has ever asked a woman who is voicing a deeply felt concern is: "Are you on your period, dear?"

When our worldview differed from that of the majority (male) culture, we were judged to be hysterical. Hippocrates (born 460 BC) opined that women became hysterical due to a wandering uterus that has been prevented from making babies. By the 1800s, women (never men) were commonly diagnosed with "hysteria" by their physicians for a variety of symptoms including a "tendency to cause trouble."

Suffragists worked on into the next century to expand women's rights and during World War II, American women gained a strong sense of their ability to succeed at "man's work." When the soldiers returned from the battlefield, these women were summarily laid off and sent back home to resume their traditional roles. Women of my generation are their daughters. We are the first of the Baby Boomers, born in the late 1940s and 1950s. Many of us continued the traditional pattern of marrying after completing high school, going directly from the parental home to the marriage bed.

In the 1960s, though, many women became determined to tear down any barrier that suggested we could survive only if some man cared for us and for our children. A steady stream of legislation expanded our rights and the advent of safe and effective birth control gave women the freedom to enjoy sex while delaying pregnancy for the first time.

This was heady stuff. Women fought to widen their career options, get equal pay for equal work, and crack the glass ceiling. Women continued to get short shrift from the medical community, which gave rise to the women's health movement in the 1960s through the influence of feminists Barbara Ehrenreich, Deirdre English, Gena Corea, and Claudia Dreifus. These women helped develop women-centered reproductive services, the Federation of Feminist Women's Health Centers, and the National Women's Health Network.

These groups noticed that women were not being included in most medical studies, and helped pass a law requiring that in 1993. Medicine's interest in developing treatments for women was overshadowed by its interest in their reproductive functions, a situation many consider unchanged today. Lack of research has left women without much gender-specific information, which implies we were not at risk for the same diseases as men.

This historic lack of information, concern, and support from the medical community is cited by Margo Maine, M.D. in *Body Wars* as reasons women minimize their own health concerns, which physicians often discount as being "in her head." Betty Freidan wrote in *The Feminine Mystique* that the medical community often ignored women's physical complaints as inevitable aging symptoms that did not require support or any form of treatment. With such attitudes from healthcare providers, it's no surprise women may ignore or deny health concerns.

Even when women do seek medical help, they often receive a different kind of care. They do not receive cardiac catheterization and bypass surgery at the same rate as men, are more likely than men to die or become disabled from heart disease, are screened less often for lung cancer, and are less likely to receive kidney transplant or dialysis.

This brief review touches on just a few of the high spots (or should we say low points) of women's self-image history. Their cultural history has taught women that they are beset by emotions they neither understand nor can control, that they are valued for their appearance and their ability to reproduce, and that someone or something else is required to save them.

Where does that leave today's intelligent, educated, energetic, and determined woman? We are going to live longer than any other generation of women has — many of us to 100 years and beyond. What do we have to worry about? Many of us are frightened of what those extra years to age 100 will entail.

MARKETING BEAUTY: WHAT IS YOUR PERSONAL BEAUTY QUOTIENT?

Researcher and educator Naomi Wolf wrote in *The Beauty Myth* that ageism still prevails and can be found in the media, greeting cards, jokes, language, and within the academic community. She said a woman's Personal Beauty Quotient largely determines her viability in the job market. The PBQ is based on a woman's attractiveness and age; it matters because it affects her opportunities for employment and advancement. This unwritten double standard means women not only continue to be paid less on the job but are held to a higher appearance standard than men. The message is, "Be beautiful and we will keep you around, but you've got to produce because you are not being paid for being beautiful."

Other feminist writers, including Carol Tavris, Marilyn French, Betty Friedan, and Dr. Maine, all attribute women's fears of aging in large part to their fears of losing beauty and value. Dr. Maine described the media bombardment of fashion, beauty, and weight reduction products to keep women looking young and beautiful. In *Spin Sisters*, former *Ladies Home Journal* editor Myrna Blyth says magazine standards of beauty and physical size are extreme and unattainable by normal women, but they want us to keep trying (and buying) "like greyhounds running around the track after the rabbit they'll never catch."

A quick glance at magazines in the grocery checkout line makes it clear that our society is possessed by a weight-loss cult that recruits young girls at an early age. Women of all ages are being diagnosed with eating disorders and most of them have been fighting negative body-image problems since they were teens. National studies indicate adolescents and young adult women make up 90 percent of the millions of Americans with eating disorders like anorexia nervosa and bulimia; these conditions affect one woman out of five.

The legendary American doll "Barbie" has it all, including a body a real girl could only achieve with extensive plastic surgery and bone removal. If the original Barbie were a live woman, she would be 5-feet 9-inches tall and would measure 36-18-33. She would be so thin she would be unable to menstruate.

. . . .

It is political because it keeps women attending to their looks instead of the circumstances of their lives.

. . . .

Women's obsession with dieting and excess weight is largely a political matter, not a medical one, says obesity expert O. Wayne Wooley. "It is political," he argues, "because it keeps women attending to their looks instead of the circumstances of their lives, it pits woman against woman, it destroys physical fitness and energy. And, saddest of all, it represents a rejection of the female body."

DOES A 16-YEAR-OLD NEED BREAST IMPLANTS?

Few issues polarize women more than plastic surgery. Most women who "have work done" do so secretly. Those who are against it scorn and condemn the women who choose to get procedures. Cosmetic surgery is one of the fastest-growing medical specialties in the United States. Considering that we live in a culture that says we are valuable primarily for our looks, and that condemns and makes us mistrust our intellect and emotions, it's a wonder cosmetic surgery isn't growing even faster than it is.

Here's our view: Women have the right to do what they want for and to themselves, and they don't need a "good excuse" like having cancer or a certain level of deformity to justify it. Every woman has a right to feel good about herself, and if that means getting a new nose, or some liposuction, that is her business. She deserves respect and compassion, not condemnation and scorn. We would especially like women to receive mentoring and support to help them build a solid foundation for their self-esteem. We talk more about this issue in Chapter 9.

WHERE ARE THE OLDER WOMEN?

If women of all ages make 85 percent of the purchasing decisions in the United States, why are older women largely invisible in advertising? Of course, ads for pharmaceuticals and ocean cruises are two exceptions. Researcher Gail Sheehy reported in *New Passages* that women were no longer aging as quickly as their mothers had, that 40 was the new 30 and that "fifty is nifty."

Friedan told us aging women could re-invent themselves over time and create a "New You." However, Peggy Orenstein wrote in *Flux* that women between the ages of 25 and 45 were very concerned about losing — not gaining — themselves, particularly about losing their youthful and sexy appearance.

But wait! Aren't women emancipated, free to choose, self-reliant, and self-assured as they age? Why are some women still unsure if their experience and knowledge can make up for not having firm thighs and flawless skin?

WHO AM I WITHOUT MY ESTROGEN?

As brilliant as the major feminist writers have been, subconscious ideas about aging and the subtle ageism still present in our culture fill many women with uncertainty and guilt. In the fairy tale, Snow White meets her downfall at the hands of a crone, a witchy, cranky old woman. Traditions like the Native American say a woman in her third phase of life (maiden, mother, and crone) should be revered as a wise teacher because of her unique intellectual and spiritual powers.

Unfortunately, few aging women today say they feel revered as crones; instead they experience ageism and discrimination. I have a good friend who never tells her age. She says, "When I tell someone my age in numbers they immediately put me in an age category: 50 = old, 60 = really old, 70 = one foot in the grave." No one wants to be categorized and discounted like that. Another friend squashes questions about her age with, "That is only relevant if we're discussing issues of age discrimination." Still another never, ever mentions her age because her husband is six years younger and she doesn't want to appear old.

I know these women are not unique. Women have lied about their age for so long they have forgotten how old they really are, and studies have shown that many people in their seventies still consider themselves middle-aged.

HOW OLD ARE YOU, REALLY?

Despite the upbeat writings of thoughtful feminists, the question that strikes fear into many women's hearts is "How old are you?" One realtor confided to me at a party, "I lied about my age for the first time today. I didn't want anyone to see me as old."

Women lie about their age and conceal the life passage of menopause because they fear it signals an end to their viability in the workplace. One career counselor advised her Fifties Woman client that menopause is a kiss of death that would end her opportunities for advancement. The recommended fix? "Just keep a box of tampons in a discreet location in your desk and that will take care of it." Women actually need much more than a box of tampons to take care of their aging issues today.

Early in my research, I interviewed Rosa, an attractive woman in her early sixties, in one of my exercise classes. I could see by the intensity in her eyes during workouts that she, like me, had the exercise-your-age-away syndrome. She said, "When I was a child, maturing women were expected to give up their girlish ways and put away stylish clothes in preparation of their matron years. Clothes defined the woman and at the age of 40, it was time to stop showing skin, cover up, and trade in those slick high-heeled shoes for boxy, sensible ones." This symbolic gesture said to the world: "I am middle-aged." Rosa hated being stereotyped and being made to dress and behave a certain way. She liked it that women who were once considered middle-aged now consider themselves vital, sexy, and full of life. But the fact is, she said, "Today we still have to fight those stereotypes by running from aging, lying about our age, and never telling anyone we have reached menopause and that hot flashes are a constant companion."

Neither approach — the boxy shoes nor the running and lying — gives a woman the space she needs to be herself. Rosa admitted it felt good to tell the truth about her fears of aging. Her words confirmed for me that I was on the right track. Perhaps my research and book might help women to lose their fears of being trapped in stereotypes. Perhaps we could talk — really talk — about our aging, our loss of youth, our changes, and our fears.

DEFINING POSITIVE AGING: CAN I STILL FEEL YOUTHFUL?

Our society offers so much information on beating the clock and staying young, but precious little on successful aging. Women who are aging well are free from the fear of aging. They are becoming the best they can be, have vibrant energy, and are ready to meet life's challenges. They regularly reinvent themselves and challenge the myths of aging. They are confident of their ability to care for themselves physically, financially, and emotionally. They do not need another person, place, or thing to make them OK. They find purpose and passion and continue to grow and give back. That doesn't mean, however, that they are immune to doubts and concerns.

We are entering an era of Timeless Women who will continue to live past 100 years, giving us time to re-invent ourselves two or three times. Many women are aging successfully, thank you very much, and having a great time doing it. Women who are aging well can continue to attain their goals and create new ones whatever their age. They are confident, independent, and self-sufficient. They are educated, know how the world works, and are not passively waiting to see what their lives will be like once their husbands retire. Instead, they are planning full and productive lives with or without a partner. These secure and confident women will make good role models for the ones who are not yet so comfortable with their aging process.

WELCOME TO WOMENSPEAK, A 1,200-WOMAN RESEARCH PROJECT

When I approached age 50, I became frustrated by the lack of useful information on women's aging. Most of the material I found fell into three types. First were the Fountain of Youth myths that denied that we had to age, as long as we took a certain supplement, followed a particular diet, or practiced the author's technique. Next were the organ and disease prescriptions, shelf after shelf, which medicalized the process of aging as if it were a disease. They focused on what can go wrong. Most distressing to me was the third type, the crone stories in which New Age authors celebrated their sags and wrinkles while mourning the loss of respect accorded to old women in our society today. None of this helped me.

Part of my interest was personal, and part was professional. As a woman, I needed reassurance. As a clinical psychologist, I needed to be able to offer guidance and assistance to clients who were experiencing difficulty with their own aging process.

I couldn't find many answers about aging in women, so I created The O'Reilly Women's Aging Inventory (TORWAI) and set out to learn more. From 1999 to 2008 more than 1,200 women answered my questions. The research results have been published for professional audiences in the June 2003 *American Journal of Health Behavior* and at an American Psychological Association annual meeting.

This section describes the survey data subjected to statistical analysis. The subsequent seven chapters expand upon that information in profiles and stories built from women's narratives, written comments, and focus group discussions. These chapters also include the strategies and tips women offered to each other as solutions to their aging challenges.

It became clear that women's ideas about aging were related to many factors: their education and employment levels, their health status, and health behaviors including exercise and dieting. Those who worried about aging were significantly more likely to diet but not more likely to exercise.

AGING BENCHMARKS: WHEN IS YOUNG?

Looking at all the answers to the questions about when certain aging benchmarks occur, women have widely varied ideas. Take age 45, for example: women variously said 45 was young, middle-aged, aged, and old.

The majority of responses did, however, show a remarkable consistency with little overlap. Most women said young is between 20 and 30; middle age is between 40 and 50; aged falls between 50 and 65; and old spans 65 to 80. It's interesting that the majority saw ages 30 to 40 as neither young nor middle-aged, so apparently we need a new benchmark.

WHEN IS A WOMAN YOUNG, MIDDLE-AGED, AGED OR OLD?

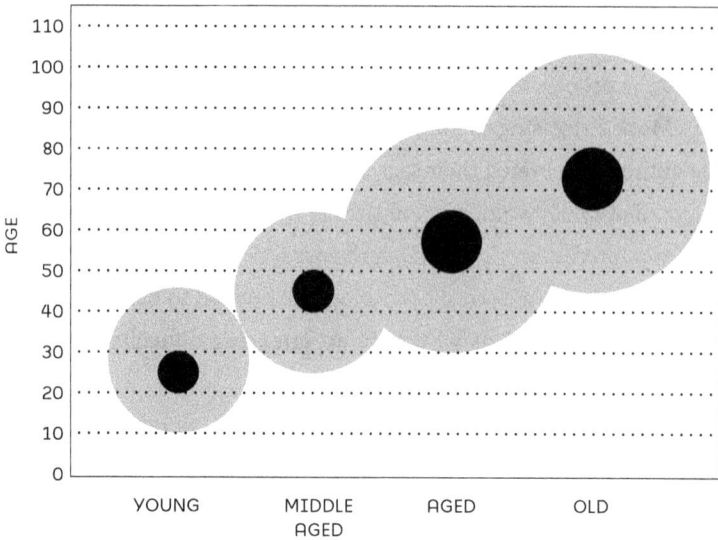

Women's ideas of age are highly variable. For example, although the majority say a woman is "young" between age 20 and 30 (the dark circle), others place the young benchmark from age 10 to forty-five. The spread increases as women get older. A woman in her forties is considered to be "young," "middle aged," "aged," or "old," depending on the point of view. Interestingly, the majority does not identify the thirties as either young or middle-aged.

....

AVERAGES ASIDE, A WOMAN'S VIEW of the aging benchmarks varies with her own age, level of education, and health status. The older the woman gets, the later she places the young, middle-aged, and aging benchmarks. Women under 50 saw young as occurring around 26; women over 50 placed it around 32 or 33. This same pattern also appeared for the middle-aged and aging benchmarks. These views are clearly relative to our own age. However, women of every age said old occurred somewhere between 70 and 80 years.

The healthiest and most educated women were significantly more likely to say that the aging benchmark occurs at a later age. Women with postgraduate educations were more likely to place the aging benchmark up to 10 years later than less-educated women. This might be because highly educated women actually live longer, enter the workforce later, and may choose to work to an older age.

Those who reported excellent health also placed the benchmark at later ages. In addition, they said middle age occurred four to five years later than those who said they had health concerns. Single women placed most aging benchmarks at an earlier age than did married or divorced women.

AFRAID OF GETTING OLDER

Amazingly, nearly half of the women — a full 45 percent — said they were afraid of getting older. Societal pressures, watching our children grow, seeing our parents age, feeling our bodies change, all remind us — every day — of the passage of time.

Fear of aging is most common in women ages 20 to 39, yet even women in their seventies are not immune. It's more common in women who are single or separated, but still affects more than 40 percent of married women. We need to face this fear because it could undermine overall health and well-being.

Only four percent of all women said they were afraid of dying. More than eleven times as many said they were afraid of getting older. Our society has provided few positive role models to help ordinary women feel confident of their own value and future as they age.

The women who were afraid of getting older tended to have more health concerns — especially abdominal problems — than those who were not afraid. They also were more concerned about their appearance, and were less confident about their ability to take care of themselves in the future.

They also told us they just don't talk about any of this. Instead, they run from it, ignore it, and have learned to keep their aging fears deeply buried.

REQUIREMENTS FOR SUCCESSFUL AGING

Why are some women more successful at aging than others, sailing easily without fear and accepting the process as a normal part of life? We received different answers from women who are afraid of aging compared to those who are not afraid. The only things both groups mentioned were role models and good health.

The women who are afraid said successful aging required things outside of themselves. Women who are not afraid believed they held the keys inside themselves.

WOMEN WHO ARE NOT AFRAID SAY SUCCESSFUL AGING REQUIRES:

....

* A strong faith in a higher power
* A good role model (mother, friend, or family member)
* A good sense of humor
* Good health
* Lots of energy
* A positive attitude toward aging

WOMEN WHO ARE AFRAID SAY SUCCESSFUL AGING REQUIRES:

....

* Having more important things to worry about
* Great role models
* Good health
* Money
* Good cosmetics
* Having a satisfying relationship
* Being surrounded by people who love her
* A happy marriage
* Having someone to grow old with

They lie about it. They hide their fears even from their closest family and friends. When Julia hit menopause early, she had no idea what was happening to her or how to cope. "It was not a happy, rose-filled adventure," Julia recalls. "It was a rocky horror show in hell." Many women also told us they would be better able to deal with it, if they could talk about it with other women and their families, and learn what to do about their unmet needs.

Women in the 20 to 29 and 30 to 39 age cohorts had the highest rate of fear of aging; after that age fear of getting older tended to decrease. Women aged 40 to 49 and 60 to 69 were the most confident in their self-care ability. Concerns about health problems and not having enough money were reported nearly three times as often as other concerns, and the patterns of concerns differed significantly by age and marital status.

HAVING A LITTLE WORK DONE

Around 10 percent of participants, 91 women, had employed some form of plastic surgery or reconstruction. Some had undergone more than one surgery, for a total of 108 procedures. Facial and breast surgeries accounted for nearly 70 percent of all cosmetic procedures, not surprising considering the attention society bestows on these attributes.

Interestingly, one of the most significant correlations in the study occurred in relationship to breast augmentation. The younger a woman perceived the young benchmark to occur, the more likely she was to have undergone breast augmentation surgery. This suggests this type of surgery may be associated with a desire to prolong one's youth.

MARRIAGE DOES MATTER

Not surprisingly, women's marital state affected their aging concerns, but not necessarily in the expected ways. Women who had never married or who were divorced rated lack of money higher than health as their aging concerns, a relationship that was reversed in married women. Single and divorced women may lack financial support and face challenges in employment including having no health insurance.

About one in ten single women expressed concern about having emotional or psychological problems, compared to one in twelve or thirteen married women. (Interestingly, divorced women seemed to have resolved their emotional or psychological problems in court. Only one in twenty-five worried about emotional or psychological problems.)

Nearly 70 percent of separated women said they were afraid of getting older, far more than single or divorced women. This could be because of the uncertainty in their temporary, separated state.

SMART HEALTHY WOMEN

Women who had more education and higher-end jobs reported having better health. Postgraduate women were most likely to report being in excellent health, whereas women having a high school or technical education were most likely to admit to having health concerns.

Women who were unemployed were far more likely to express concerns for their health than those in professional or technical jobs. It was not clear why: Did the unemployed have active health problems that contributed to their unemployment? Were they primarily concerned about a lack of employer health insurance?

Health Risks: Time to Take Your Own Temperature

Denial is queen. Most women could not identify any specific health concerns, probably because they tend to put others' needs first: "This can't be a heart attack — I've got to take care of my family!" While Dr. Mom's loving touch wipes the tears from little cheeks and bandages a host of scrapes and cuts, who is taking care of her? Did she get a mammogram this year?

Health rises to first place in aging concerns by age 30 and stays there until age 69. What is especially troubling about this trend is although women say health is their greatest aging concern, most don't identify any specific health issues they are concerned about. This suggests they are not taking necessary preventive measures.

Women Would Rather Diet Than Exercise

Interestingly, worries about getting older do not necessarily prompt women to do the things most likely to improve their health. Those who worried about getting older were significantly more likely to diet but not more likely than non-worriers to exercise regularly. This was also true of women who were worried about their ability to care for themselves and their problems 20 years hence.

About half of the women said they exercised regularly, generally three or four times a week. Those who perceived aging as occurring earlier were more likely to exercise, while those who perceived it to occur later were more likely to diet.

Dieting: Ruled By Your Thin Person

Weight management is a huge industry in America and it has become a way of life, particularly for women. We have Weight Watchers, Jenny Craig, Sonoma Diet, Cheater's Diet, Flavor Point Diet, Supermarket Diet, Longevity Diet, South Beach Diet, French Women Don't Get Fat, Eat Right 4 Your Type, Dr. Atkins "New" Diet, 3-Hour Diet, Dr. Phil's Ultimate Weight Solution, Zone Diet, Raw Food Diet, Sugar Busters," and "Lose 10 Pounds in Three Days" diets, and name-less crash diets, just to name a few.

Social researchers have noted that women's repeated exposure to unrealistic images of beauty in the media drives them to pursue an impossible body type. Women often equate being thin with staying young. This is great for business, but it's really bad news for women's self-esteem and body image. It is especially troubling to see that women's concerns about their ability to age successfully may be subverted into dieting rather than into behaviors that might more positively affect their aging process.

Only six percent of women we surveyed mentioned their weight as their major aging concern, but more than half of the women said they monitor eating habits to control their weight and 36 percent of women said they diet. Women with health concerns were significantly less likely to monitor their eating habits than women who reported excellent health. Only three percent said they used exercise to manage their weight.

For women's long-term success at aging, it is especially troublesome that those who do worry about aging tend to diet rather than exercise. This might indicate that these women regard their weight as an appearance issue rather than a health issue. Whatever the reason, this is an unbalanced strategy because both diet and exercise are essential for long-term health. In fact, a National Institute on Aging study showed that exercise confers more health benefits than dieting does.

Many women seem to have "bought" the cultural message that weight loss is their answer to total mental and physical health. When we asked many women what they did to feel good about themselves, they said, "Lose weight." Although maintaining a healthy weight is essential, it cannot take the place of exercise and practices targeted to a woman's specific health risks.

Exercise And Buns Of Steel

National studies have shown that around 60 percent of women exercise regularly, which was approximately what our group did, although this varied by age, education, and employment. Women in the 30 to 40 age group exercised the least of any age group (around 40 percent) and women in the 70-plus age group exercised the most (75 percent). Younger women involved in childcare and taking care of families may have limited personal freedom. Older women have more time and may have learned the benefits of exercise and staying healthy. The higher the level of education, the more exercise the woman incorporates into her life, but marital status was unrelated to frequency of exercise. Two-thirds of women in excellent health said they exercised regularly compared to less than half of those who said they had health concerns. Interestingly, fewer than one-third of women of average health said they exercised regularly.

Health Risks: Don't Tell Me

Our results confirm that many women may misperceive their health risks for the most common causes of death and disability. Fewer than four percent of participants mentioned concerns about the two leading causes of death for women: heart disease and cancer. Not one mentioned a concern about AIDS, Alzheimer's, urinary incontinence, or mental illnesses including major depression, anxiety, and phobic disorders, although these conditions are common in women. This disregard of health concerns may have tremendous impact on women as they get older because it may prevent them from employing preventive measures. Women seem to blithely ignore their health risks, perhaps because they are so busy taking care of the needs of others.

Although it might not be surprising that respondents younger than 40 ignore health threats that may not manifest for another 20 or 30 years, nearly half of the participants were over 40 and one-fourth were over 50.

FINANCES: SHOW ME THE MONEY

Concern about finances tops the list for women under 30 and is consistently the top aging concern for at least one in four women of any age. Women usually earn less than men, and only partly because they take time off to raise families. Women need to get comfortable finding better paying jobs, learning to manage their own money, and meeting their own financial needs.

WOMEN OF EVERY AGE

Women's aging concerns took different priority order in the different age groups, but the top four concerns were consistent across all age groups. Women in the different age cohorts have different life experiences and needs, so naturally their concerns reflect their changing priorities.

We did not seek to survey women under age 20 although a number of them completed surveys online. Looking informally at a small number of responses, we noted that these very young women were afraid of being alone, rejected, and unloved, often felt confused, and were wanting to find acceptance and a place in society. Primary concerns of women under age 20 were lack of a mate, being alone, fear of dying, and a loss of psychological well-being. In fact, with the exception of not having a mate, which was mentioned most often by the 70-plus group, no other age cohort expressed so high a rate of concern for these factors.

Some were already fearful of losing their youthful looks and were feeling the marketplace pressure to match up to idealized images in the media. They are trying on various ideas of what it means to be a woman. We also know from other research that these very young women are particularly vulnerable to eating disorders and body image difficulties, which if untreated may persist throughout their lives.

TWENTIES: IT IS TIME TO TAKE ME SERIOUSLY

Between ages 20 and 29, women's aging fears of not having enough money increased by nearly half, exceeding the rate of any other age cohort. Fear of having health problems increased over the teenagers by a similarly large jump, beginning a fairly steep climb that peaks in the sixties. Concerns about not having a mate and fear of dying dropped by more than 60 percent.

Nearly 60 percent of women ages 20 to 29 also said they were afraid of getting older. Twenty-something women confront a whirlwind of choices surrounding their educations, independence, income, career, debt, friends, a mate, and starting their own families.

THIRTIES: I AM REALLY A WOMAN NOW

Respondents between ages 30 and 39 reported a dramatic 77 percent increase in health concerns. Concerns about loss of psychological and emotional well-being, however, dropped 63 percent compared to those of women in their twenties. Other concerns changed only slightly compared to the younger group.

Thirties Women are working on the balancing acts that most will continue to perfect throughout their lives. They strive to keep some sense of their own boundaries while they juggle key tasks associated with their jobs, career paths, mating, and finding stable relationships, all with an ear to the ticking of that biological clock.

FORTIES: I AM RUNNING OUT OF ESTROGEN

Between the ages of 40 and 49, women's concerns were quite similar to those of women in their thirties. The one notable exception was that fear of dying dropped by more than half.

Forties Women felt time accelerating and most feel ambivalent about their age. They have begun to develop patterns of self-care and look forward to the emptying of their nests. They are still concerned about relationships and family but now are remembering their personal needs and interests apart from their families. Many reconnect with their spouses to rekindle love and passion, and most of them become more determined than ever to spend quality time with their women friends.

FIFTIES: I AM AN AMAZING CREATURE AND YOU'D BETTER NOTICE

In their fifties, women's responses were similar to those of women in their forties. However, concern about health problems, which dropped slightly in the forties, rose again. Concern about being alone and losing youthful appearance, never reported very frequently, dropped further; however this trend was not significant.

Nearly half of women ages 50 to 59 were afraid of getting older. Everyone comments that their outside appearance no longer matches the way they feel inside. Some felt sadness, but not everyone is particularly distressed by this development.

Fifties Women re-evaluate their lives, their jobs, and their relationships, and were making changes in pursuit of greater satisfaction. Passion and purpose begin to figure in the Fifties Woman's vocabulary and they are finding their voices like never before. "I am woman, hear me roar," could be the theme song of the Fifties.

SIXTY: TIME FOR ME AT LAST AND YOU CAN JUST WAIT

Noticeable changes occurred between women in their fifties and women in their sixties. Fears of not having enough money dropped by a third, and fear of having a spiritual void — never very high — dropped by two-thirds.

A large national survey found that nearly half of people ages 65 to 69 considered themselves to be "middle-aged." They still don't *feel* old at all — until they glimpse themselves in the mirror.

Sixties Women are self-assured and less susceptible to the influences of advertising in the marketplace. They trust in their intellect and life experience and are ready to say, "Move over world, it's time for me!" Their high rate of concern for their health leads many of them to improve their nutrition and exercise programs and to take better care of themselves. Many also were rediscovering their sexuality and finding ways to present themselves to their partners and the world as super-sexy women.

SEVENTIES: I WANNA DANCE AND KICK UP MY HEELS AND I WILL

Change from the sixties to the seventies showed a more than quadrupling of concern about not having a mate (interestingly, this was not matched by a corresponding increase in concern about being alone). In addition, concern about health problems dropped precipitously by 64 percent to approach the teenage low. Even though they are feeling the aches and pains of aging, they have for the most part adapted and feel they know what to expect. Overall, most were healthy and active and wanting to find their purpose and passion. Re-inventing themselves was very much a discussion.

They wanted to be able to care for themselves and finances were a strong consideration. Many of these women expected to have long and productive lives, a love interest, and plenty of new projects and ways to contribute. What thoroughly annoyed them was being perceived as too old to be interesting. Most of all, they wanted respect.

EIGHTIES: MAYBE I WILL MAKE IT TO 100! WANNA COME TO MY PARTY?

Eighties Women were surprised to find themselves actually this old. They surprised us as well with the vibrancy and interest they felt for their lives. These women understood that aging was real but still expected to live fully, be active, go to the gym, play golf, date, and give back to the world. They were seasoned women with much to offer. Many wanted to mentor other young women and were giving back by helping younger women get ahead. They were using all their knowledge and love of life to help others. Driving and staying independent of course was a huge issue. All of these women had grown up caring for others and did not like the idea of burdening others with their care. They had few regrets.

TALKING ABOUT AGING DOESN'T HAVE TO BE SCARY

We have only just begun our journey and we would like to share what other women have told us. They wanted us to know how they felt and what was working and what was not working for them. Most women have entertained some if not all of these thoughts.

This book is for all the women ages 20 to 100 who want to feel youthful at any age and who plan on living past the age of 50. We are writing for those who are concerned about the emotional, psychological, and physical impacts of aging, and who care about their daughters and granddaughters and want to help them age well, too.

The women's profiles in this book are composites of real women ages 20 to 89. My professional experiences with women in more than 20 years of clinical practice have shaped this book, and it includes the words of the generous women who shared their views. It is our privilege and opportunity to share their thoughts and concerns.

The raw material for each chapter was the responses of women within a single 10-year age cohort (say, twenties, thirties). We gathered these stories from the surveys, from seven large focus groups, and from e-mails and comments at my speaking engagements, and from our combined 120 years of experiences as women.

The profiles reflect women's reality in proportions that reflect statistical reality. Some women in our profiles fear aging, others do not. They are single, married, divorced, remarried, or widowed. They are mothers and they are childless. They have focused on family, home, or career and every imaginable combination. They have fears to express and advice to share.

One of the most exciting things about writing this book has been seeing that the women's stories become richer and richer in detail, perspective, wisdom, emotion, and experience as they get older. Our reviewers tell us they recognize themselves on nearly every page. This book is about women's truths, and some of them are telling us they have a ways to go, even though they have survived a lot since the days of the menopause tent. There is so much we can share and learn from one another.

Certainly, we have come a long way, yet we have a long way to go when it comes to having comfort and security as we get older. It's an economic fact of life in our society. Our feminist "mamas" identified women's concern with body image and staying young and not becoming invisible. They discussed the way women allow societal pressures to control the fashions they wear and the weight they should maintain to be accepted. They suggested women are being pressured to have unwanted cosmetic surgeries. That's fine as far as it goes, but the Women-Speak Project wants to help women regain their faith in themselves and in their own abilities to care for themselves. We want to help them find peace of mind with their minds, their bodies, and most of all their souls.

We affirm every woman's right to feel any way she wants and do anything she wants for herself. We are here for the women who are feeling bad and having problems with this aging thing.

We Want This Book to Help Women:

- Stay healthy and productive
- Acknowledge health risks and act to prevent illness
- Counteract feeling invisible
- Rejoice in the power and wonder of women
- Help women be informed, cared for, and to thrive
- Use their voices to help themselves and others
- Feel youthful at any age

CHAPTER 2 *The* **20s**
Fearfully Young and Glowing

I am not a child anymore and I want to be taken seriously.
JANIE, 21

Twenties Women find themselves thrilled — and terrified — to be "grown up" at last, more or less on their own, with the reins in hand, and facing life's many challenges. They've got a lot of issues to think about (education, jobs, serious relationships, marriages for some, starting families, and more responsibilities than they have ever had to contend with). The twenties age group is by far the most diverse age group we surveyed and talked with. One Twenties Woman was trying to combine a job with a new baby, another was just trying to finish her education; all were contemplating their next moves. Many of these women reported feeling overwhelmed with the rapid-fire emotional and psychological changes they experienced. Growing up and being considered an adult was the ultimate job description for many of these women. They knew they had a lot to learn and also felt they had plenty of time to master these new issues.

Indeed, a Twenties Woman can expect to live a long time. Those who celebrate their twenty-first birthdays today can expect to live *at least* another 60 years to become 81. Many will live much longer. They will likely have several careers and re-invent themselves numerous times. Twenties Women confront major life changes at every turn: completing their educations, establishing their independence, beginning to earn an income, developing a career, paying off student loans, finding their niche in a circle of acquaintances, selecting a mate, and starting a family. Most of them feel anxious about being adequately prepared. They are working hard to build confidence in their own abilities. Having fun is still a priority, and those who aren't already exhausted from tending babies will often stay up all night with friends just for fun.

The massive self-consciousness and anxiety of their teens ("Is my dress cool? Is he looking at me?") has given way to a greater focus on performance. Feelings of inadequacy still fuel their questioning: "Am I the person I should be? Are my parents proud of me? Am I letting others down?" Not yet far from their teens, they still ride an emotional roller coaster. Psychological issues are still common in Twenties Women as they work to develop a healthy self-esteem and self-image.

Many life passages occur during the twenties. Census data tell us that half of women who marry do so for the first time before age 25. One-third to one-half of women who become mothers will birth their first child by age 25, and nearly 10 percent of women have already divorced by age 30. Twenties Women notice that their perspective changes as they begin to reach milestones they once regarded as terribly old, notably age 30.

WHAT TWENTIES WOMEN WORRY ABOUT

With all the challenges they face, it's no surprise nearly 60 percent express a fear of getting older, half again more than in women under 18. Perhaps because so many years stretch ahead of them, Twenties Women have the greatest fear of getting older of any group. It's not because they are silly, shallow, or unintelligent. Far from it.

As for their aging concerns, Twenties Women worry equally about death, family, friends, and kids. As parental support wanes, their concerns about money and health increase. They worry more about family, perhaps partly because they see their own parents aging, and partly because they are thinking about establishing their own families. In a decade or two, Twenties Women will take their place in a new, sandwiched generation that will scramble to care for themselves, their parents, and their children.

Meanwhile, Twenties Women overflow with youthful energy and hope for their future, which makes them more confident in their future ability to care for themselves than any other group. Boomer parents have worked hard to instill positive self-esteem, with the unintended result that some Twenties Women may have unrealistic expectations about how easily and quickly they will advance in the world.

Twenties Women imagine (in most cases erroneously) that their futures will be less stressful than the present and that they will have fewer things to juggle. In truth, demands on their time are likely to continue to increase for several decades.

Twenties Women feel most successful as they master the externals: a decent job, maintaining physical fitness, and repayment of educational debt. Other marks of social success are having a solid social network and good relationships with parents. Building successful relationships with other women and men is a primary focus and they feel more confident when older women share their strategies and experiences to help them to better understand the prospect of growing older. It's interesting that even things that others might regard as failures, such as a divorce or becoming a single parent, carry a large measure of satisfaction. Twenties Women may think, "At least I have successfully accomplished this rite of passage."

This chapter tells the composite stories of Jessica, Melissa, Stephanie, and Amanda as they discover their roles in relationships and in community. They rise to the challenges of taking responsibility for their own homes, jobs, and families. At this early stage of their journey, they experience excitement and anxiety in equal measure.

JESSICA: "I WAS BARELY RESPONSIBLE FOR MYSELF, THEN SUDDENLY RESPONSIBLE FOR SOMEONE ELSE."

Jessica, 23, is afraid of getting older. She married at 19 and became a mother before she was 20, neither of which she had planned. She recently divorced her ne'er-do-well abuser husband. As a teenaged mother she had to grow up quickly, so she never got to experience the playful twenties. With her needy infant to care for, she did not have the luxury of an extended and self-centered youth.

"Having a child created ten times the emotions I was not prepared for," Jessica says. "I was barely responsible for myself, then suddenly responsible for someone else." Her teenaged concerns about parties, vacations, and fun quickly gave way to coping with a colicky baby, childcare, divorce, and figuring out how to succeed as a working mother. Looking back, she wistfully remembers her teen years as the last time her own needs topped her to-do list. She has had to focus her energies outside of herself, and time has become her most valuable commodity.

Early on she learned to accept the fact that single motherhood at such a young age — for all its rewards — limits her ability to fulfill other dreams. "I wake up in the night and wonder: 'How will my life change?'" Jessica says. "Will I be prepared for those changes?"

"To me, success means my child is healthy and happy," Jessica says. "Although I work, my real career is raising my child." She was not prepared for the ferocity of her love. She would lay down her life for him.

Jessica's parents are divorced, but they remain united in their support and without their help she would be in big trouble. "I truly appreciate my parents for who they are," she says. "As a mother myself, I have gained respect and appreciation for what they have given me. As I make progress toward getting a better job and supporting myself, I'm so grateful for the huge role they have played in my development."

She quit school to marry before she completed her college degree. When her shotgun marriage went bad, she went to beauty school and became a cosmetologist so she could support herself fairly quickly. However, in some weeks her earnings barely cover the cost of childcare. Although she knows of a position that would pay better, having a flexible schedule so she can care for her son is her top priority. Although she is working to complete her degree, she can take only one or two classes per semester, and even that leaves her exhausted.

Aging looks like a much scarier process now than when she was younger. "I looked forward to getting older as a child, but now I'm afraid of it," she says. She often feels overwhelmed and struggles alone with her fears. Her women clients at the salon scare her with their gossiping. She's scared her parents will die, and that her son will die. "And I don't want to talk or think about any of it," she says.

Although many women use their youth and freshness to get attention, Jessica downplays it. "People think I am too young to be taken seriously," she says. "A young woman is not seen as intelligent."

Even so, Jessica cares a lot about her looks. She is one of 10 percent of Twenties Women whose mantra could be: "Stay young and beautiful if you want to be loved." She weeps when she catches a glimpse of herself, uncombed, un-bathed, cradling a sick child, and struggling to keep her life together. Sometimes she chokes with anger at herself and resentment of her circumstances.

Leaving a first marriage changes a Twenties Woman's relationship priorities. "If a woman is not a mother at 20, I guess she would worry mostly about her career or petty boyfriend-girlfriend problems," says Jessica. "My concerns at age 23 are stability and caring for my child. I worry about providing for my child and making a good home life.

"I really think that aging would be easier with a committed and supportive marriage partner," she says. It's hard work being alone, and Jessica dreams of finding "the perfect man and then not ever have to worry about splitting up."

Instead of fun, excitement, and romance, Jessica's priorities now include "a healthy and trusting relationship that I can rely on," and her past experience leads her now to proceed with caution. "All women are vulnerable to getting hurt by men and other women." Her definition of "the perfect man" has changed drastically from her teens, when it did not occur to her that some kinds of relationships could actually be far worse than having *no* relationship at all. "I want to feel that my opinion is valued and that I am loved," she says. "It takes finding a mature mate with goals, one who can provide attention, understanding, and faithfulness."

For Jessica, women in their thirties or forties are unimaginably older than herself. Like other Twenties Women, she wants to create her own definition of aging, to decide how she fits into society, and to determine for herself when—and whether—she would ever be considered *old*.

"One day I realized my parents were getting older. I'm the baby and all my older brothers except one disrespected them. I try to respect my mom and dad after I made a conscious choice of role model—who did I want to be like—my brothers or my parents?

"I think my mom handled getting older pretty well," Jessica says. "She told me the hardest birthday she faced was her thirtieth. Now as she gets older, she talks about how young she still is instead of how old she is. She says we have to go along with what God has planned for us. My other role models are my grandmother and my co-workers. At the salon I work with a lot of women around my mom's age, so I get to watch them face getting older."

Jessica sees clearly that society's attitude toward aging is negative. "Society puts way too much emphasis on age for determining our importance to people," Jessica says. "The older the woman, the less importance our society places on her, and the less respect people have for you. I think old women are beautiful! My mother is 57 and the most gorgeous woman alive! She's single, too, and because I have to care for my child, I can't be there for her as much as I think I should."

Despite her fears, Jessica wants, "to get all I can out of life and not waste a moment of it. I wish that I would stop aging and get more money to get more schooling. And I wish that I could find a man who would not leave me for a younger woman simply because I age. And I hope that I would be able to really learn from the mistakes I've made."

. . . .

JESSICA IS A TWENTIES WOMAN with a great many strengths. In her limited number of years she has become responsible and realistic about her roles and doing a good job as a mother is important to her. She also is determined to get ahead in life. Ending an abusive relationship was a wise decision so that she and her infant would not spend another moment in a relationship that would place them in harm's way. Many young women stay in toxic relationships because they are afraid to be alone and fear they can't care for themselves or their children as single parents.

Jessica recognizes the value of her parents as a resource; they both help her make good choices and feel supported. Parents who are committed to assisting their daughters and grandchildren keep many young single mothers and children out of poverty and off the roller coaster of social services. Jessica is focused and on track to achieve her goal of independence and is willing to work as long and as hard as is necessary to meet her goals. Women who accept their responsibilities and quickly learn the skills they need can face their futures with hope and confidence.

One challenge that Jessica will have to face sooner or later is that she has missed out on some key steps necessary for her to become a mature, responsible adult. She looks enviously at the girls her age who are dating, going to parties, traveling, or trying out different jobs without pressure. Ready or not, young single mothers miss the trying-out period and step directly into adult responsibilities. Like Jessica, they worry about their futures and the changes in their appearance. Their party days are over, especially since they often cannot relate to other Twenties Women who don't understand the seriousness of their responsibilities. They need to find ways to understand both their personal needs and how to fulfill them.

Jessica feels regret for the choices she has made as well as guilt for the consequences that her parents and son must share. Working with a counselor or support group may help a young mother devote enough attention to herself so that she will not become resentful of her circumstances. She may need emotional and psychological counseling to cope with the stress surrounding her double duties as a single parent and a working student. Her greatest obstacle will be to find respite time to rejuvenate and find friends with whom she can socialize. Twenties Women need their friends to provide important peer support, to share childcare, and to help them develop good patterns of diet, exercise, and mental health.

Although Jessica has a positive role model for aging in her mom, whom she loves and considers beautiful, she needs to examine her choice of an abusive mate. Women who grow up in a disrespectful household often have a hard time establishing their personal boundaries. Unless they devote conscious attention to changing their expectations, they may choose one abusive man after another. When they can learn to consciously make better choices, they have more energy available to pursue what they really want in their lives. Once they are clear they can focus on acquiring the training and skills they need to improve their marketability in the workplace and achieve financial and emotional security.

Jessica faces the additional challenge of trying to match up to society's standards of beauty. Her work in the beauty industry intensifies this, and she listens all day to the criticism and cattiness that women heap upon other women, which escalates her fears. On the other hand, Jessica is ready to be taken seriously as a professional and hates the way her co-workers and bosses tease her and patronize her youth. Being called a "cute little thing" absolutely enrages her and strengthens her determination to be able to earn a grown-up wage and take care of herself and her boy.

MELISSA: "I'M STARTING TO WONDER IF I'LL FIND A RELATIONSHIP THAT IS SOLID."

Melissa, 29, is lively and popular. She has dated a lot, and although she has entered into two serious long-term relationships since college, she is still single. Although she thinks often about getting older, the process doesn't scare her. "When I was a teenager, I always wanted to be older; 18 was the *magic age* I always wanted to be. Now, I take my age in stride and enjoy the perks and challenges of each year as it comes. I don't think about getting older any more often than the rest of my friends do.

"I don't *think* old," she says. "But it's funny because when I was 20, I thought 30 was old, and now I'm going to *be* 30. I wonder if people think I look 30 because I don't feel like I look 30.

"I'm starting to wonder if I will find a relationship that is solid," she says. "To be honest, I think *a lot* about the fact that I am single and nowhere close to being married, or finding the person I want to marry.

"When I was younger, I thought I had to be married young, and so I never really planned for single life. When I graduated college as a single woman, it was a little scary. But I took it one step at a time. I completed my master's degree and began my career, and have made the best out of life."

Still, what she looks forward to most is having a family. She goes out with friends, is active in her church, and has even tried blind dates and some Internet services, with no luck so far. Lately, she has been buying and filling her apartment with commercial photographs of adorable babies in cute costumes. "It bothers me that I still won't be married by the time I'm 30, and that I'll still be scraping by. My financial priority is paying off my student debt, and saving."

Melissa has thought a lot about her future and has developed a to-do list for getting older: create financial security, buy health insurance, exercise and eat healthy, develop good relationships with God, family and friends, and remain involved in her church. She feels like she has those things under control.

"My one concern is I just don't want my body to give out," she says. "I want to be able to do the things I do now forever. I wonder if I'll be healthy in my older age." She has no particular health issues yet, though, so she rarely visits a doctor.

"I think of my age most when I go home to be with my family and when my single friends and I get together. The topic of being single in my late twenties always comes up. My friends and I also discuss the fact that we don't feel as old as we actually are.

"It helps to discuss my feelings with my single friends, because we have a lot of the same feelings. We crack jokes about it, and find humor in the situations we find ourselves in. I'm not the only one that feels invisible when I'm with a group of couple-friends, or when my girlfriends are discussing their wedding plans.

"When the worrying gets to me, I tell myself that I'm still young, and that I should enjoy my single life while I can and make the most out of it. Sometimes I'll go work out if I start to get too stressed out." Overall, though, Melissa takes a positive view and tries to stay in the present rather than thinking of her future. "You can dwell on the negative or you can move on," she says philosophically.

"I look at the positive side of things and try not to worry too much," she says. "Oh yes, I admit I did start coloring my hair, and I've gotten my eyebrows waxed," she says with a laugh. As for most other Twenties Women, her body feels strong and capable, so her priorities focus more on her clothing, weight and muscle tone, haircut, and teeth than on worrying about things like possible heart disease or cancer.

Like other Twenties Women, Melissa wants to find meaning in her work. "A helping profession lets you get more out of work than 'just a job.' You can walk away from it and feel good about yourself," she says. She's always been very self-directed, confident, and able to make her plan and work it. "I just followed from step one without any detours, whereas others go with the flow with many changes."

After completing a criminology degree, Melissa took a job as a firefighter and trainer. She loves it, but says, "There's a near-total lack of women in the male-oriented firefighting field. I can really see my male colleagues banding together to get their way at work," she says, "And they try to derail me by saying I'm, 'sleeping my way to the top' or 'a lesbian.'"

She respects the board of directors and chain of command at the fire department. However, even though everyone knows that gender discrimination is clearly illegal, she says, "It's awkward to have to go against the chief. If you go to the board with a complaint, you're putting yourself out there. You sacrifice yourself even if it is the right thing to do." She swallows a lot without comment because she wants to advance in her career, and because in such a complex work environment, she finds it hard to trust herself about what to do.

Melissa bemoans the lack of successful older women mentors who are happy with themselves. She had a college professor who was a great mentor but has not found anyone to confide in since joining the fire department. "It's difficult to pave the way when you don't know how. I'd like to mentor other women myself," she says. In her free time, Melissa also volunteers, teaching literacy and English as a second language. "I love knowing that I can help others, and make a difference in peoples' lives."

Although she loves the challenges of her career, she says, "I would love to stop when I have children, so I can be a stay-at-home mom. If that won't be possible, then I'd like to work from home or part time when my kids are little. The determining factor will be income. Once my kids are all in school, though, I'd like to go back to the fire department."

Of course this plan hinges on finding a daddy for those kids, "someone who will not pass judgment on my actions and will listen well, and wants to have a good time," Melissa says. "It's about being loved for who I am, finding a man who fits my ideal of mankind. I want someone I can live with the rest of my life, someone sexy who can make me happy." She is not about to let go of that dream but if she finds herself still unmarried as she approaches age 35, she has decided to use a sperm donor to have a child or adopt on her own.

Unlike most Twenties Women, Melissa can look ahead and glimpse retirement; for most it seems impossibly far off. "As far as what age I'd like to quit working, I haven't really thought that out yet, although I'd probably want to retire by 55 or 60," says Melissa. "Maybe I could if I have good saving practices and assuming the city keeps funding our pension plan. I don't know if I'll have enough money, though, because I don't think I can get my Social Security money until I'm like 67.

"I don't really mind getting old because 60 isn't even considered old anymore," says Melissa. "But then I think about my parents who are only 53. My mother told me 'It's all downhill after 50,' but my feelings are totally different from hers. She acts old, and she has lots of back, neck, and sinus problems. I tell them all the time they're not old and they need to stop acting like it. I hope to never act old.

"Reaching 50 was a big issue for my mother," Melissa continues. "She worries about getting older and about my future, probably more than I let her express. I'd rather try to be optimistic about it." In this Melissa says she chooses to be more like her grandmother. "She is 80 and does whatever she wants and is proud of it."

....

I can't wait to be really old — like 80 — so that
I can be a #@&%)! and everyone will blame it
on my being old.

....

Melissa agrees women are judged on their looks rather than their intelligence, and she's always felt embarrassed by not being pretty. Even so, like most Twenties Women, she emerged from her self-critical teens with a clear view of her best features. "I love having a good smile," says Melissa. "And I want to look fit. I'm not skinny — I would have to work too hard for that — but I want to be able to keep up with everyone."

Even more important, she says, "I wish to never lose my brain power. My intellect and my ability to think are what make me unique and keep me whole. The rest is just bonus. And I don't want to take any age for granted. I want to appreciate myself and my life at any age, not yearn for it later when it's gone. I want to find eternal satisfaction with who I am, and become wise enough to enjoy my age and my appearance."

The most important factor in getting older is, she says, "Staying true to who I am, because if I can't stay true to myself and be real with myself, then I can't be real with others." Melissa thinks the automatic valuing of youth and looking young or trying to act young is awful, though she understands the pressures to do so.

"My friends perceive me as 'ballsy,' so my advice is to grow some balls! This *is* all about *you*. This is your life. Stop thinking about aging!" she commands. "Think about how you're living your life. Are you happy? Are you living your dreams? Are you making the most of your life? Stop for a minute and consider the alternatives to growing older: would you rather die young without ever fulfilling your dreams and leave nothing for others to remember you by? For heavens sake, you start aging at birth! Why worry about it when other people call you ma'am or open doors? They are just being nice."

For women who feel devalued as they get older, her prescription is simple and emphatic: "Reject that value system!" she says. "Think of Sean Connery, David Niven, and other sexy older men, and train yourself to see older women with the same respect and admiration! Don't get tunnel vision. Let original outside thoughts creep in and see women for who they really are."

. . . .

MELISSA IS EXCEPTIONALLY SECURE FOR a Twenties Woman. She is capable, self-made, and self-assured, realistic about her goals, and financially self-sufficient. Her good planning skills enable her to keep necessary things in place such as financial stability, health insurance, and being able to care for herself no matter what happens. Twenties Women like Melissa have a positive attitude and set goals for themselves with confidence. They are not afraid to be challenged and are open to new and exciting possibilities.

Although she yearns to have a husband who will enable her to be a stay-at-home mom, she does not let the absence of "Mr. Right" get her down. She feels she is about to enter a new era with her thirtieth birthday, and is giving herself another five years to find a mate. After that, she is prepared to take her desire for motherhood into her own hands. She has too many hopes and dreams to sit back and let her life run on autopilot. Melissa has a positive, realistic attitude about her prospects and is determined to be successful at whatever she does. She has every reason to succeed.

Women today feel comfortable choosing single motherhood when they have not found a life partner but wish to have children. They can gain ready access to information in support groups and through the Internet about how single motherhood might affect their lives and careers. A good support system of friends and family helps women whether the stresses associated with this decision and the sharing helps them feel they can handle whatever life brings. Overall, though, Melissa's youth still prevails over her concerns about getting older, and she copes mostly by laughing and having a good time with her girlfriends.

Melissa's challenges include making sure she will be financially and emotionally able to care for herself and a family without having a mate. The idea of not having children may leave a woman feeling sad and incomplete and lead her to choose to go it alone. When they can keep an upbeat attitude and continue to seek more from their life experiences and relationships, single women like Melissa can go on with their lives with great zest.

Women who choose so-called non-traditional roles may encounter identity issues and develop negative self-images. Melissa's work in a male-dominated field has raised a more perplexing question: "Must I be more like a man or can I still act like a woman in a typically male occupation?" It's not surprising that Melissa's image for being assertive is to become less female and more male by 'growing balls.' Melissa needs to find ways to assert her boundaries and rights without compromising her female identity. The conflict Melissa feels to be tough and do her job and at the same time to act more like a *traditional* female is a problem that women of all ages must resolve if they are to excel in nontraditional careers.

What she wants to do, and what makes her feel successful, may be seen as inappropriate by her coworkers and family members. Melissa needs to understand how her profession and her career are affecting her social and personal life.

She needs to find as much information as possible about her job choices before she tries to make a career change.

If both men and women give Melissa negative feedback about who she is because of her career choice, she may feel very alone and misunderstood. Mothers continue to be a primary role model for their daughters. Melissa appreciates — almost envies — the freedom she sees in older women as well as their openness. She really likes their willingness to share their views about being a woman and their determination to be true to themselves, but she struggles with the lack of female mentors in her chosen field. If Melissa would join a national association, it would open up her world and help her find other female firefighters to learn what it takes to have a successful career and a good family life.

Melissa does understand the importance of taking care of herself. The physical demands of her job require her to work out regularly to maintain her strength and stamina. She knows she needs financial fitness as well. She is completely clear that her parents are no longer going to take care of these issues and the men she has met were *certainly* not going to do it either. The responsibility is hers alone, and she has started early in planning for her financial, emotional, and physical well-being. Melissa uses her workouts to manage her stress, has developed good self-care habits, and serves as a good role model for other women.

STEPHANIE: "WHENEVER I POSE A THREAT TO MY BOSS, SHE OBSTRUCTS ME."

Two years ago, Stephanie, 26, married a wonderful man who shares her values and goals. She is thrilled by the intensity of emotions that wash over her: love, passion, joy, and a deep satisfaction that this is the right path for her. Her husband is 11 years older than she, which she realizes raises a potential problem for her later in life. "I don't want to become a widow but recognize that with our age difference it's likely at some point," she says.

Stephanie's focus lies primarily on her relationships with other people, and like other Twenties Women who already have committed partners, she especially wants to keep the relationship strong. "Love and life is the way of happiness," says Stephanie. "Cherish the days that you have with your mate, for if he is happy, you will be happy.

"I hope that we will live a full, long life," says Stephanie, "and that my husband and I will die together. I hope to always surround myself with people I love and can learn from and reciprocate with throughout my life." She looks forward to having new experiences and gaining wisdom, and to traveling more on the job and with her husband.

Although she delights in her marriage, she resents the way older family members and friends pressure her with the question, "When are you going to start a family?" She has known since her teens that she will not be able to conceive a child and that is fine with her. Her husband has children from a first marriage and neither one of them is interested in adoption.

Stephanie is on staff at a service agency for people with developmental disabilities, where she thinks the older women employees must perceive her as a threat. Although there has been an obvious increase in the amount of money raised after she was hired, she experiences subtle psychological abuse from her female boss who holds her back and takes all the credit. The top boss is male and Stephanie sees her female boss as "getting away with everything. It's an ongoing battle: What should I say, when should I keep my mouth shut?"

They have never established a good rapport and Stephanie is at a loss how to repair the poor relationship. "Whenever I pose a threat to her, she obstructs me," Stephanie says. "She didn't even invite me to the Christmas party! But I see her agenda and I refuse to let my boss control me." This lack of trust makes each workday unpleasantly tense.

A major challenge for Twenties Women is finding their niche — at work, in society, in their circle of acquaintances — and dealing with bitchy women poses a common challenge for young women who care so much what others think of them. "You can put bounds on it, though," Stephanie says. "It's possible to talk about others without being mean and gossipy. Talking about friends with people who also know and care about them is not bad-mouthing. But when people outside the circle do it, that's meanness and you'll get a reputation for having a big mouth. I definitely choose not to be with such people."

As happy as she is in her new marriage, the prospect of getting old truly frightens her. "I wish society would view older women as the mature, intelligent, beautiful people they are," says Stephanie, "but it doesn't! We have to compete, and I think good skin care is a key. The world today is very hard on women of all ages."

Always very attractive, Stephanie values physical appearance highly, both for herself and her spouse. Talking with her grandparents, seeing their health problems, preparing a resume, or planning for her future can all trigger her fearful thoughts. "It bothers me to see TV commercials that talk about women in their twenties showing signs of aging. And I know that the products are cleverly marketed towards my fears."

Her mom has never really talked much about aging other than to laugh about it. "She doesn't even dye her graying hair," Stephanie says. "I don't believe she thinks much about it. She'll joke about her saggy breasts, but that's about it. She says 'It happens ... deal with it, and be happy to have your health above all else.'

"I try to be like my mom, but the idea of looking old just freaks me out," she says. To regain her calm, Stephanie tells herself: "Everyone goes through this, and I am at an advantage over many people because of the support I have from friends and family and the good choices I have made and am making." Part of those good choices is the good self-care she practices. "I'm very fit and lean now, but I put on weight easily and always have to watch my weight," she says. "I don't look at it as a bother, though; regular exercise is just something I have to do. The alternative (being heavy and out of shape) is not an option for me. I like myself now; I don't want to think about having wrinkles or saggy breasts."

Your body is an instrument. Don't think of it as just an ornament.

Occasionally Stephanie has felt she's too young to be taken seriously on the job, a problem that is compounded by the fact that she is petite. A lot of the people she meets within corporate fundraising are middle-aged men. If they get into a confrontation or she disagrees, they don't like it and will try to shake her confidence with remarks about her youthful appearance or her age, like "Where's your hall pass?"

Because she's tired of such put-downs, she does look forward to being recognized as a woman, not a girl. After all, she is taking a mature approach to her preparations for getting older. She exercises regularly, maintains her appearance, plans for her financial future, and nurtures her relationships.

Stephanie worries about being hurt by today's economy. She has no faith in the American healthcare system, and believes the country's social network is disintegrating. "I'm afraid that our savings won't be worth much. Social Security will be non-existent by the time I retire, and it's hard to predict how much I will need to live on. I'd love to retire at 65, but I'd have to have enough money to do so first."

Twenties Women are still gaining a sense of who they are, and the basis for their self-image is primarily external and a bit vague. "It's important to me to feel successful and be happy and present a confident image of myself. Knowing I'm a bright, attractive, and well-liked person is so important to me and I hope to always have great people in my life who love me for who I am. Of course I've got to keep my personal integrity."

Stephanie's husband was married to someone else when they met and although she doesn't think much about it consciously, she does wonder sometimes, "Will my mate stay with me?" She feels guilty about the pain she caused his ex-wife, and has also watched two friends endure the heartbreak of rejection, one by a long-term boyfriend, the other by a new husband.

Aside from her guilt, her greatest concern now is her health. "Since I sit in an office for nine hours a day, I worry about bone/joint issues more than anything. And of course knowing that my parents will eventually pass is hard to swallow."

But those models are hard to find. "Wouldn't it be great to have different TV programs about the wisdom of the older members of our society?" Stephanie says. "And how about commercials portraying older people using the products and doing the same things the rest of us do? When I see how older women are marginalized, I feel really uneasy about getting older myself."

. . . .

STEPHANIE'S STRENGTHS GIVE HER A wonderful foundation to help develop her own personal power. Deeply perceptive women like Stephanie know what they want. If they have been fortunate enough to find the love of their lives, they feel complete and they are happy with the way things are. Stephanie wants to avoid change in her personal life and gets frustrated when she feels pressure about starting a family so she resists all the unwritten social rules they expect her to follow. Women are often recruited early into the caregiver role, and Stephanie is not even aware that she has readily accepted responsibility for her much-older husband's health. She is already worrying if she is doing enough to keep him healthy and alive. Her fear of being left alone adds to her anxieties.

Stephanie wishes she could adopt her mother's view of aging but appearance is much too important to her. Her mother's priorities are to be happy, to keep her good health, and to ignore social pressures to stay young and beautiful. Although Stephanie admires the older woman's confidence, she does not share it. Knowing the media manipulate their fears does not necessarily keep women from buying into the messages that they need to look young at all costs. Women like Stephanie feel confused by society's expectations. Even though they may reject a social requirement such as producing children, they may still be unable to fend off the perception that aging will somehow take away their self-esteem.

Stephanie's mother is clearly a good role model of successful aging, and it's unusual for a daughter with such a model to be so fearful about losing her looks. Like so many women her age, Stephanie has been taught since girlhood that she must "stay young and beautiful" to stay loved.

At this early stage of her life Stephanie already has several worries beyond losing her looks: not having enough money, losing her health, and becoming a widow. A woman with an older husband needs to discuss his health needs and put a plan in place for the time that his health might fail or he might die. It's important to be realistic about a large age difference and develop a financial plan that will allow comfort and security. Saving and planning relieves women's anxieties about their futures and long-term care insurance is especially affordable when one is young. It is never too early to plan; it makes for better sleep each night.

Women also need to attend to their own health. Even a woman like Stephanie who has always been healthy, and who both looks and feels great, needs to have regular medical check-ups. These should include a mammogram if she is at higher than normal risk for developing breast cancer and other screenings tailored to her history and situation.

She worked hard to complete her degree and now Stephanie wants to advance her career. Although most Twenties Women haven't been in the workplace long enough to bump up against the glass ceiling, they may feel held back by other women. Stephanie and her peers have never known a world without lightning-fast communications and they expect to live and advance at a fast pace. When older women speak of the overt discrimination they have encountered in the workplace, Twenties Women listen with disbelief. They expect equal opportunity and advancement as their due, especially when they enter a workplace that already has many women in management.

Instead, they are shocked to feel obstructed and un-mentored by older women in the workplace, and may even find some men more willing to help them advance than the women. They expect immediate credit and recognition for what they do and may believe they should be able to compete directly with their managers. What is Stephanie thinking? *Of course her boss obstructs her when she feels threatened!* Stephanie may erroneously attribute the obstruction she feels to bitchiness on the part of the other woman rather than perceiving the age-old corporate dynamic in which the boss (regardless of gender) takes the credit. In this model, underlings have a better chance of advancing if they focus on making their boss (regardless of gender) look good. Although most women managers actually receive higher ratings on collaboration in the workplace, that is certainly not true for all of them, and most will not tolerate someone who overtly tries to outshine them.

Twenties Women definitely need someone to guide them in the ways of the working world if they are to avoid an endless self-defeating cycle of disappointment. They also should find someone with whom they can talk openly about their concerns about their looks, careers, and ability to care for themselves. A career coach, counselor, or even a support group can help these young women feel more successful as they age.

When they are feeling calm, women like Stephanie look forward to gaining the respect and knowledge they believe will come with getting older. In some ways, they are excited about growing older because they believe they will be taken more seriously. Stephanie admires the life her mother leads as an older woman and envies her happiness and openness to friends and acquaintances. Even fearful women like Stephanie can learn that it is possible to age successfully. Women who become comfortable with themselves can let go of their dependence on their looks. They can learn not to care so much what society thinks and stop rating themselves using their sex appeal as a guide. Stephanie can listen and learn from her mom's positive view of aging and they will feel closer to each other after they have talked about the source of their ideas about aging.

In order for fearful Twenties Women to truly believe and live by their egalitarian ideals, they need to spend more time with peers who have different values and with older women they admire—maybe Fifties and Sixties Women—that they see as being successful and intelligent without being nipped and tucked by plastic surgery. If they associate with older women who are happy and aging success-fully, they may better accept their own maturing process.

AMANDA: "I'M AFRAID THAT WHEN I'M OLD I WILL REALIZE I DIDN'T ACHIEVE ALL I HOPED."

Amanda, 21, really enjoys her job designing and setting up displays in a retail store. She relishes the opportunity to use her artistic talents, but her wages have barely paid the bills. With regret she's returning to her former job as a waitress in a dinner house where she dislikes the job but earns good tips.

"I wish I had a better job," she says wistfully. "Career-wise I'd like to do some-thing meaningful that would make a difference. Maybe later, when things are less stressful and I have fewer things to juggle."

Amanda moved out of her mother's house at age 17 because they fought constantly. "I have a very difficult relationship with my mother. I wish she would back off. I love her but I disagree with her on everything, so I chose my own path."

During her difficult adolescence with her controlling mother, Amanda learned to conceal her feelings. Now she has a hard time revealing them, or for that matter, even noticing what her feelings are. She keeps herself emotionally covered and protected.

"There are not a lot of female mentors in my family and it's always been hard for me to find female friends. I distance myself from them because I've had so many bad experiences. You know the type of girl who always has to create drama, always needs to put someone outside the circle. It's exhausting! I have lots of guy friends, but I don't trust other women and keep them outside."

Amanda judges other women harshly and turns the same critical eye on herself. She once thought she wanted to become an artist, and took every art course offered at a local junior college. But her mother ridiculed her goals and pressured her to go into business. Ultimately she dropped out; she couldn't make herself take the other courses needed to graduate.

"I'm afraid that when I'm old I will realize I didn't achieve all I hoped," she says. "In school my counselors and teachers went on and on about completing things in a certain time frame. Then all the peer and family pressure about college — it had to be the four-year plan or the five-year plan. I couldn't do it. I hate it, but I still worry a lot and compare myself. I think, 'I'm 21, so I should be done with school by next year,' or 'I should have a baby by the time I'm 25.' So what if it takes me longer to decide what I want to do?

"I worry that I'll work so hard to get somewhere and do something and then hate it," Amanda says. "You can't know in your freshman year what you want to major in. I couldn't wait to get out of college; now I wish I could go back. Part of me is scared to go back to school, plus I don't see that their degrees did my friends much good. Maybe part of the value is learning what you don't want to do."

Although she doesn't usually look very far into the future, she does hope to gain more knowledge and intelligence along the way. "At the moment, I wish I were older. I hate to think I'll always feel this uncertain and confused," she says.

"At this point, I just want to live fully in this moment and be happy with myself," says Amanda. "I wish that I will always find joy in life and will never become downtrodden. Age is in the mind. Physically speaking, I try to care for myself, but I had friends who died at 17. What is the sense of fearing death? It is only rebirth."

·······························

I try to look at age as a beautiful thing,
the older the wiser.

·······························

Amanda had her first serious boyfriend when she was nearly 20, but that didn't last long. "I don't think a woman needs much from a relationship at this age, because I think 21 is too young to be getting serious," says Amanda. "The most important thing is, she shouldn't sleep around. Really, my friends and I are thinking about things like, 'Can I get enough money to buy my own car? Do I have money for gas? Do I have a date for this weekend? For tonight? What do I wear? What do people think of me? What do they think of my home?'"

Amanda sees herself as completely unique and she can't imagine her life in future decades with any detail. "I doubt my needs at age 30, 40, and so on will be the same as anyone else's," says Amanda, "and I doubt they would change if I were with a different person. Once you've grown up, a woman's needs won't change," she says. "The only change would be personal needs for each of us as individuals."

"Society and the media should stop pressuring and promoting women's looks, because that causes disorders, depression, and deaths," says Amanda, who feels strongly about this issue. "Look at our models in magazines. They look starved. What is that telling younger girls as they grow up? Only a tiny percent of women actually look like that. People need to stop and look at the person on the inside and not the outside. Looks are not everything, and people do age, some faster than others. It's a fact of life and men do it also. There needs to be more respect for the aging adult. Society needs to quit centering around the young because you're only young a short period of time."

Amanda gives herself credit for the myriad adolescent fears she has already overcome: going through puberty, finding a first boyfriend, learning to drive, getting into college. "Having a supportive group of friends really helps," Amanda says, "but really, just experiencing things, like the college application process, forces you to get over fears."

For all her uncertainties, Amanda is not afraid of getting older and sees things differently from fearful Twenties Women. "Women age successfully by being happy with themselves and their relationships," she says. "Being too worried about what's going on just adds stress to your life, and you can't be happy. Women should stop reading *Cosmo* and the other magazines that make us fear growing old. All those ads for age-defying make-up make us covet youth, but it's not reality. Aging is natural and something to be looked upon kindly. With age you gain experience, understanding, and wisdom even though our culture puts a much higher value on firm breasts and tight asses."

She's read a lot of feminist blogs on the Internet and believes that self-esteem is the most essential foundation for successful aging. "Having a positive self-concept and self-esteem is the most important factor for a successful aging experience," Amanda maintains. "You have to have a sense of humor about yourself, you can't take yourself too seriously." It's pointless to obsess about losing a younger self, she cautions. "We need to realize that we are continuations of the same selves at any age. Yes, we change as a result of our cumulative experiences, but our core being remains fixed. Don't listen to what others say, listen to yourself. By dealing honestly with ourselves now, we can help to contribute to a better aging process."

. . . .

AMANDA PERCEIVES HERSELF AS A strong woman; she is very much determined to become her own person, self-reliant, freethinking, and independent. Young women who leave their birth families early have to grow up quickly and find strategies that allow them to make sense of the world. They gain support from their friends even though many young women display a disappointing lack of depth and an under-developed self-concept. Women like Amanda feel they are in charge of their decisions and that is one of their great strengths. They are proud to find their own way and scorn other women who are too worried and concerned about their looks.

A young woman's feelings of inadequacy and confusion have complicated roots, often in their troubled relationships with and rejection of a very conformist mother. As young girls they were given approval for being pretty and sweet and given every beautiful and materialistic Barbie doll toy. The message was pretty clear-cut. When they become adolescents and rebel against this female model they receive a different message. In no uncertain terms the message says, "You are *not* OK" and "You'd better get it together." When a mother's behavior sends a strong message that a woman's looks are her most important attribute, young women may feel angry and determined not to let such societal pressures have any place in their lives. In fact, Amanda's mother is obsessed with remaining thin, so Amanda has put on a lot of weight and neglected her appearance to prove there is more to her than her looks.

One challenge young women like Amanda need to overcome is their perception that they do not need a good education. While they may find a path that does not require a college degree, most young people today cripple themselves if they do not acquire one. When they eventually realize they want to rise higher than entry-level jobs, they often return to school. Fortunately Amanda does understand that she has a lot to learn, is patiently granting herself time to learn and grow. Meanwhile, she is determined to enjoy where she is right now. Her talents and artistic flair sustain her and she is able to keep herself motivated even though her own mother has discouraged her from pursuing her dream.

Amanda feels her plate is full just living day to day. Pressured by society and family to grow up, finish their education, decide who and what they are, women like Amanda become confused and overwhelmed and just check out. They never stop resenting and resisting this type of external pressure.

When women have a difficult time with trust they need to find someone to exemplify positive ways of coping and living. Without positive role models they have no idea of what it is to be a successful Twenties Woman, so it is difficult for them to develop a healthy self-esteem and self-image. As they try on different roles and concepts of being a woman they benefit from positive mentoring from peers and older women. One huge roadblock to this learning is the subtle, undercover way that women compete and undermine each other. Amanda mistrusts other women because she does not know how to handle this covert competition. She covers up her insecurity with a know-it-all attitude that makes it almost impossible for her to ask for or receive help.

Amanda spends a lot of time wishing, yet has so far been unable to take focused action for her future. Women like Amanda do not perceive that they are still making choices to spite their mothers. If they are unable to come to some peace and understanding about Mom, they may remain confused and frustrated; some professional counseling can help them understand the tasks ahead of them as they mature. Twenties Women who have few positive life experiences have a hard time developing a feeling of trust, which blocks their ability to learn from others. Their fierce independence isolates them from family, peers, and support systems, all elements that are crucial to personal development. With a professional to help them sort through their trust issues, intelligent and talented young women like Amanda can develop the positive self-esteem and self-image that allow greater happiness and personal satisfaction.

NORMAL DEVELOPMENTAL TASKS FOR TWENTIES WOMEN

- Choosing a mate
- Achieving a feminine social role
- Learning to live with a life partner
- Birthing children
- Rearing children
- Managing a home
- Getting started in gainful employment
- Taking on community responsibility
- Finding a comfortable social group

HEALTH TIPS FOR TWENTIES WOMEN

. . . .

- ❧ Take part in enjoyable exercise
- ❧ Eat fruits and veggies
- ❧ Wear a seatbelt
- ❧ Get regular health screenings from ob/gyns and family practitioners
- ❧ Practice safe sex and protect yourself from STDs
- ❧ Find healthy relationships and get out of abusive or toxic relationships
- ❧ Find ways to relax (yoga, tai chi, meditation, deep breathing)

WHAT DO TWENTIES WOMEN WANT?

Most women of every age will say that age 25 is *young* and many say the years between 25 and 35 are the best — the most desirable — of a woman's life. Some of this nostalgia surely stems from forgetting the reality of the Twenties. Twenties Women are beset with anxieties and concerns and have a greater fear of getting older than any older age group.

Women in their twenties have many concerns, notably the financial burdens of the steadily increasing cost of living, competition for well-paying jobs, large student loans, and a softening economy all make it hard for these women to feel confident about their ability to take care of themselves. Twenties Women are just starting on the normal developmental tasks of adulthood, which probably accounts for their being so fearful and anxious about caring for themselves.

Most Twenties Women have an external focus, thinking of career, family, cars, possessions, and homes rather than their personal character or spiritual development. Preparing for getting older is the furthest thing from most of their minds; their horizons are only as close as finding a decent job and trying to stay in shape. As with all women, the simple process of living their lives will eventually bring greater understanding of their strengths and weaknesses. Paradoxically, while Twenties Women fear aging more than any other group, they also seem to have the most knowledge, information, and resources available to help them with aging issues and fears.

Twenties Women who are afraid of getting older express their concerns differently from those who are not afraid. This difference in expression actually carries through all age groups. Those who were afraid of getting older expressed their aging concerns in passive terms, citing things like "loss of independence, being useless" and "How will I be treated?" These fearful women worried about physical deterioration, and in particular about losing their mental capacities.

In comparison, women who were not afraid of getting older used much more active language to express their aging concerns. They are afraid of different things, things that reflect their sense of self-efficacy, such as "not accomplishing all my goals, be happy with myself, unable to achieve all I wanted, and succumbing to the will of others."

Nearly every Twenties Woman we surveyed expressed wishes about growing older and these wishes reveal a lot about their worldviews. One overwhelming difference between fearful and fearless women was that ten times as many fearful ones as fearless ones wished to slow down the aging process. They wished "To never grow old, to be 23 forever, to stop aging." These wishes show up in fearful women of every age who are sensitive and react strongly to media pressure to stay young and beautiful. Fearful women were also much more likely to wish for happiness, contentment, or enjoyment of life.

RESPONSIBLE FOR HER OWN HEALTH?

Unless they have chronic conditions, most Twenties Women take for granted their young, strong bodies. Many do not yet perceive health as something they must create for themselves. Women today rarely die in childbirth, and better nutrition combined with medical miracles should keep these women alive and well longer than those in previous generations. Women are in the process of deciding what to do with all of that precious time.

The health concerns of Twenties Women center on their reproductive and sexual functions, a focus reinforced by society's interest in them as breeders. Their concerns include the side effects of birth control, miscarriage, infertility, abnormal ovulation, cervical cancer, and endometriosis. A few have high cholesterol and high blood pressure, but none mention a concern about heart disease. Many mention stress- and lifestyle-related issues. Although many Twenties Women are sexually active, none mentioned a concern about sexually transmitted diseases.

Some Twenties Women had multiple complaints, like Melissa's friend Beth, who lists "asthma, bursitis, eczema, gastrointestinal disease, bad circulation, and

STEPS TO FINANCIAL RESPONSIBILITY

. . . .

* Learn to budget and save each week

* Take advantage of any profit sharing or investment possibilities on the job

* Stay out of debt, limit yourself to one credit card, and pay off debt each month

* Attend investment meetings and learn about finances

* Start investing early with whatever you can spare: $5 a day at a 9 percent return (assuming we ever get back to that rate):

  ~ in 20 years becomes $100,000

  ~ in 35 years becomes $440,000

  ~ from age 22 until retirement at 65, becomes a million dollars

see sidebar next page

overweight." She adds, "My doctor seems to think that my problems are because I'm a girl." This is a terrible message for young women to receive from the medical world, especially because many of these conditions might well respond to a healthier program of nutrition and physical training. Many in the medical community still see women primarily as baby-makers, which removes their human dignity and reduces them to their reproductive functions.

It is tragic that so many young women do not realize the importance of healthy lifestyle choices for prevention of chronic conditions like cancer, heart disease, and diabetes. Many do not understand the difference between dieting to achieve a societal ideal of thinness and eating in a way that allows them to achieve and maintain a healthy weight. Although they may fit into a size 2, they may have starved themselves into undernourished weakness and ill health.

We hear their suspicion that consequences may follow in comments like: "I hope that in five years I am still active, healthy, and as happy as I am right now. I hope that my current lifestyle choices don't have too great an impact on later lifestyle choices. I'm trying to exercise more and eat healthier so I can continue to age (gracefully of course)!"

Although some physicians say young women don't need mammograms, the truth is that women in their twenties and thirties are being diagnosed with breast cancer every day. If a woman knows she is at increased risk — or if her intuition tells her to get checked — by all means she should insist on being screened. Guidelines are just that; they are not hard and fast rules. Many women can benefit from earlier initiation of screening and they must learn early on to advocate for their healthcare needs.

Twenties Women — like the women in every age group — seemed largely unaware that the leading cause of death for women, as for men, is heart disease. By developing healthy lifestyles now, Twenties Women have an opportunity to prevent the development of disease and they may very well live to see cures developed for breast cancer, heart disease, stroke, and other major killers.

MONEY TO LIVE ON

The financial concerns of Twenties Women often focus on the short term: paying off educational debt and trying to make the transition from school to adult life. College students often work at least part time. Although the gender wage gap has decreased in recent decades, women still generally earn less than men, and the wage disparity grows wider as they get older. Today, fewer and fewer jobs provide good retirement plans. In most cases, education is a key to advancement and greater earning power, which often comes with so-called nontraditional jobs.

The medical community has noted a nationwide trend. In 1966, just seven percent of medical school graduates were women. In 2005, 47 percent were female. If this growth continues, it is conceivable that some day, female physicians will provide the majority of services. This is changing the idea that medicine is a nontraditional job for women.

My ob/gyn is a mother with two small children and she wants to be seen as a working mother who provides excellent service to her patients; however,

STEPS TO FINANCIAL RESPONSIBILITY

- Find a mentor to help with your finances and learn as much as you can
- Give to others who are less fortunate
- Take business classes— understanding what it takes to run a business will help you succeed as an employee or employer
- Visit WIFE.org for more ideas

KEYS TO HEALTHY EMOTIONS

. . . .

❧ Get help for recurring feelings of anxiety and depression, feeling helpless and hopeless, or feeling powerless or overwhelmed by life stressors

❧ Notice the signs of stress, such as insomnia, changes in eating, and being unable to relax or concentrate—do something to manage stress before long-term problems arise

❧ Hormonal imbalances can occur, so talk to your doctor if you feel out of whack

❧ Build your relationships based upon mutual respect and consideration and they will give you comfort and help you feel good about yourself

see sidebar next page

she also wants her hospital employer to remember that she is a working *mother* and it is not her intention to work the hardest nor to be away from her children for long hours. For our society to truly embrace family values, businesses will need to change. Women want and need to work, but not at the expense of our families. Like firefighter Stephanie's, some career paths are still inhospitable to women.

When asked what they look forward to about getting older, some Twenties Women talk about retirement, being able to relax, and doing volunteer work, and most don't expect to wait until they're 65, either. That age just seems too far off. Others take a shorter view and focus on aging milestones they will encounter sooner: the joys of career, settling down, having children, and traveling. Some see pregnancy as offering a Baby Break in their working years and most have not considered — or do not care about — the cost to their careers.

. . . .

Growing older is a gift from God. Tomorrow is not promised to anyone. If you make it through to see another day, be grateful and live life to the fullest.

. . . .

SEEKING LIFE GUIDANCE

Because aging appears as such a fearsome prospect to so many Twenties Women, many are frustrated by a lack of healthy successful older women to serve as good role models and mentors, particularly in the workplace. It would be worthwhile for them to focus their energies on identifying and finding a female mentor. In fact, many companies are developing programs to help women advance in the workplace. In today's corporations, hiring from within is increasingly important to stop the high costs of turnover and to keep good employees from walking out the door.

Mentoring helps young women learn strategies that help them succeed, and forms an important resource because the popular media offer precious little advice or guidance beyond fashion, makeup, and how to stay sexy. Naturally such tips are inadequate for making the transition from being a *young woman* to becoming a *grown woman*. Many do not feel prepared and find the transition mysterious and confusing.

Twenties Women are metaphorically trying on so many different hats that they feel overwhelmed by all the decisions they must make. A few generations ago, they perceived few options beyond marriage and family. The historic pattern through the 1950s had most women traveling in their teens or twenties from their parents' home to the marriage bed where they would birth 3.2 children. Although this pattern has undergone many changes, women still feel a societal pressure to have marriage, children, and a successful husband.

Women today do have many more choices about what they will do with their lives. For example, today's Twenties Women often entertain nontraditional views of marriage and having children. Although their biological clocks are beginning to tick more loudly as they near the end of their twenties, some of them plan to skip marriage or children

KEYS TO HEALTHY EMOTIONS

. . . .

- ❧ Balanced diets and regular meals are essential for health and emotional well-being—if you know someone with an eating disorder, urge her to get help now

- ❧ If you are having a problem it is not a sign of weakness to seek outside help or information

- ❧ Staying connected to good support systems is key to emotional health—do not isolate yourself

EMOTIONS OF
TWENTIES WOMEN
. . . .

- ❧ Fear of aging and losing the look of youth
- ❧ Fear of emotional illness due to anxiety
- ❧ Excitement about new freedoms
- ❧ Feeling overwhelmed by new responsibilities
- ❧ Confusion over changing roles and responsiblities
- ❧ Desire to find a partner
- ❧ Yearning to have fun and be happy
- ❧ Anxiety about ability to care for self
- ❧ Worried about what others think
- ❧ Desiring approval and acceptance
- ❧ Excitement about a career and gaining independence

entirely, or they may intend to marry and reproduce much later in life. Many consider staying single an attractive option.

Historically, women have always worked, many as sole providers or, more often, providing essential supplementary income for their families. However, Twenties Women today usually *expect* to work before — and often after — they have children. Another change from earlier generations is their perception of living in a dangerous world. Theirs has been called the Endangered Generation because they have grown up in an unsafe world full of drugs, guns, and violence.

While they are experimenting with relationships, most Twenties Women date a number of potential partners. Most of what they learn, of course, is about what they don't want and what doesn't work for them. Near the end of the twenties, most women get tired of looking and want to settle down, but wise women hold out for compatibility of values, attraction, sexuality, and spirituality rather than just settling for an available candidate.

CREATING A HEALTHY EMOTIONAL LIFE

Women's attitudes toward aging, specifically their fears, definitely affect the way they view their futures. We found that Twenties Women who are afraid of getting older were much more likely than less fearful women to mention wanting a relationship at all. They also much more often described their desired mate in generic, unqualified terms such as "a mate, someone, a boyfriend, marriage" rather than listing some qualifying characteristic. Young women who are not afraid of getting older tended to qualify their image; not just anyone would do.

They wanted: "The right person, the perfect mate, someone who truly loves me, a mate to be satisfied with for the rest of my life, that special one, a good man, or someone who shares my interests."

Although it's common to think of young women as being more frivolous and fun-loving than their elders, less than one-tenth of Twenties Women listed "fun" as an important relationship concern. Instead, they were interested in "attracting the cutest guy and having a great time with him, making sure everybody thinks they look good, and going to parties." Less than half that many mentioned sex as important to a relationship.

Unless they are already mothers, Twenties Women make little mention of children other than in an occasional theoretical reference to "having babies." Their focus is on first things first: finding a mate. If they are single mothers, they have identified that they want to find a mate who is stable, who will stay with them and help raise the children. Single mothers in their twenties make up some of the lowest paid workers in the United States, which leaves them and their children extremely vulnerable to a lifetime of poverty.

Twenties Women see their mothers' attitudes pretty clearly. After all, their mothers are Baby Boomers who have little difficulty expressing themselves, but differences in age and experience prevent their daughters from feeling a sense of commonality. Most of the Twenties Women said their feelings were probably similar to their mothers' even though they didn't identify closely with the same issues. They also are aware that their generation did not have the same financial or educational challenges as

TWENTIES WOMEN WANT OTHERS TO KNOW

- ❧ I am intelligent and I have much to offer
- ❧ Take me seriously and teach me what you want me to know
- ❧ I am passionate about my life and what I can offer the world
- ❧ I am afraid I will not be able to live the life I want
- ❧ I worry I will not find a mate, have children, and be happy
- ❧ I get confused about what I want and what others seem to want for me
- ❧ I am eager to find my path and I need mentors to guide me
- ❧ I want friends and people I can trust and with whom I can be myself

see sidebar next page

TWENTIES WOMEN WANT OTHERS TO KNOW

. . . .

- ❀ I don't understand how to handle women who compete in negative ways
- ❀ I have so many dreams and want them all to come true
- ❀ I get overwhelmed with all my new responsibilities and just want to be a "kid" again

their mothers and other role models, and hence were not able to relate. Many Twenties Women are entering the working world for the first time, competing for jobs and salaries with older women and men. Although women overall still receive lower pay than men for equal work, most of these young women do not expect to encounter this problem.

Twenties Women are still learning what it is like to be themselves, so they are still trying to bring images of themselves into clear focus. They are smart and thoughtful about their ideals, however. They want to please and fit into their society and families, yet they also want to remain individuals who make a difference.

They have witnessed women's rebellion against the prevailing shallow beauty culture and may consciously reject it. Even so, many Twenties Women — like women in every age group — expressed some level of dissatisfaction with their bodies. This reflects the fact that our society has become possessed by a weight-loss cult that recruits girls at a very young age, even in infancy. Eating disorders are rampant, affecting an estimated one-tenth to one-fifth of young women.

. . . .

When a man speaks,
people listen, then look. When a
woman speaks, people look, and if
they like what they see, they listen.

. . . .

Some feminist observers say women's obsession with dieting and weight is largely a political matter. Because this obsession keeps women working on their looks instead of trying to change the actual circumstances of their lives, it puts women in competition with each other. The focus on appearance destroys their physical fitness and energy, and sadly, leads them to reject their own bodies.

This is tragic for the women themselves, but for young women, many of whom will become mothers, this can have dire consequences for their babies as well. Some young mothers are so pre-occupied with weight gain that they risk their unborn infant's health with excessive dieting while they are pregnant. A large study has found that many new parents don't understand that "baby fat" is necessary for growth and is essential for brain and nervous system development. Well-meaning parents may start their children on the diet treadmill and ultimately set their pre-adolescent girls on the path to becoming future anorexics.

A primary task for the Twenties Woman is to develop a positive self-image and reinforce her sense of self. Two key types of awareness will prove invaluable. First is to become aware of *catastrophic* thinking, such as, "I will die, I will be in an accident, I will lose everyone I love, I will never find someone to love me." These thoughts immobilize a woman. In contrast, substituting positive self-statements frees a woman to act on her own behalf.

The second skill is to become aware of *crystal ball* thinking. This is thinking that suggests you can predict the future: "If I do this it will be the end of my world. If I upset him he will leave me." This is not realistic thinking because no one can see into the future. In fact this type of thinking may help attract the very outcome most feared.

REINFORCING YOUR SENSE OF SELF

- Positive self-esteem, positive self-image, and a realistic body image are keys to successful living as a unique individual

- Find positive role models and mentors to help you chart out your life and career

- Make each day the very best you can and begin each day with a mantra: "I am special. I am unique. My presence makes the world a better place."

- Connect with a higher power or philosophy and seek peace in that relationship

- Accept yourself and give yourself credit for what you are—you make a difference

- Give of yourself and you will never feel alone

GET RID OF STINKEN THINKEN: IT'S MAKING YOU CRAZY!

. . . .

* You really can overcome denial, lack of confidence, and excessive worry about the opinions of others.

* Get rid of toxic people in your life who bring you down. Instead, surround yourself with people that make you laugh and feel good about yourself.

* Replace negative self-statements with positive statements such as, "I have a strong healthy body, I have beautiful eyes, or I am very good at math."

* Worrying is a bad habit that you can break. Write down what you are worried about. Are these worries real or imagined? What is the point of your worry? Choose to do something else with the time you spend worrying. Give your worries away.

see sidebar next page

If a woman is still struggling after using the tips on the Stinken Thinken checklist, she should consider finding a professional to help her examine what she wants. There is no weakness in asking for help and a local mental health association will be able to make a referral.

The bottom line for Twenties Women is to keep a healthy outlook on life, which includes acceptance of what will come their way. Try to view growing older as an accomplishment, much the way some women view pregnancy's stretch marks as a medal marking a successful life passage. It's so important to take good care of oneself and stay in tune with one's body to be physically well, without obsessing over the little signs of aging.

In order to build their spirits and self-esteem, Twenties Women often reach for something outside themselves. They say they feel good when they receive validation of their ideas by others, compliments on their appearance from friends or professors, good grades, a satisfying love life, and good times with family or friends. Very few mentioned making themselves feel good by doing things *for themselves*, such as exercise, preparing a healthy meal, or even going to the beach.

LOOKING FORWARD TO GETTING OLDER

"Being older will be great!" is the overriding message from many Twenties Women who look forward optimistically to maturing. Despite their many anxieties and fears, they have big plans and expect many positive things to come with greater age: more experience, stronger relationships, more knowledge, more respect, less concerns for other's opinions, more internal resources, less susceptibility to romantic turmoil. They expect to acquire a greater ability to see things clearly rather than believing the surface presentation, and to understand what things are truly valuable. They want to log more memories, meet more people, know themselves better, have more time once they retire, and have more financial security.

Dr. Nancy's Kick-Butt Keys for Twenties Women

- Get your body moving. You will feel great.
- Get rid of all the 'shoulds' in your life.
- Learn to say no to the things in your life that make you feel bad and yes to things that make you feel good.
- Surround yourself with positive people. The laws of attraction really do work. If it makes you feel good about yourself then it is the right path to take.
- Expect to be happy and expect to have the best life possible.
- Learn something new each day and never stop learning and growing.
- Find your passion and purpose. Giving to others: this is a supreme way of being fully in this world.
- Stay up-to-date in your job skills and learn to sell yourself to your boss.
- Travel and try new things.
- If you feel invisible or dismissed do something about it.
- Find a mentor and learn as much from her as you can.
- Live, love, and laugh a lot to feel great.
- Give yourself credit for being an amazing person.

GET RID OF STINKEN THINKEN: IT'S MAKING YOU CRAZY!

- Become aware of the negative self-statements you say to yourself, such as, "I am fat, I am ugly, or I am not smart."
- If you worry about your looks, exercise is the best way to change your attitude and feel better about yourself. Exercise produces happy hormones (endorphins) that make us feel good.
- If you have a negative attitude, get out and challenge yourself with something different: take a drawing class, learn a new language, travel, join a hiking club.
- Visit the Help Yourself section at WomenSpeak.com for information about relationships, finance, health, and growing older.
- Be nice to yourself and expect others to do the same.

Twenties Women accurately perceive that their futures hold much excitement and many rewards. As older women will tell us, all the expectations that Twenties Women hold can be met and they will in large part create their own lives in line with these expectations.

We leave the Twenties Women at the golden age of 29, viewed by some as the last desirable birthday to acknowledge. It's an old joke: "Please come to my annual twenty-ninth birthday party."

The anxieties so many Twenties Women face about finding a job and a mate will be replaced by babies, growing families, and figuring out how to succeed at what they have worked so hard to become: working mothers. Others sidestep motherhood for a while—or permanently—to focus on careers, personal goals, or helping older family members. Looking back from the thirties, they may regard their twenties wistfully as the last time their own needs topped the to-do list. Moving into their thirties, women reach ever farther and they find themselves juggling more plates in the air.

Visit www.womenspeak.com to learn more about the twenties. Express yourself and share ways you have learned, grown, and found your best life.

CHAPTER 3

The **3Os**
A Great Balancing Act

I never thought it would be like this. I feel like I'm standing
on my pinkie toes trying to keep 30 plates in the air.

KIMBERLY, 35

Thirties Women are perfecting their balancing acts. As they drive from work to family to community to soccer field and back, they may find themselves searching the crowd for their own faces. I'm busy and happy, but exactly where am *I* in all this? Delighted as they are to finally be fully adult, in their free moments they puzzle over myriad questions. As they marry and form new friendships they wonder "Do my old friends still fit in my life today?"

Birthing and guiding their children consumes untold hours and they barely have time to wonder as they crash into sleep: "What will my life be like *after* my kids? Who am I now? What's happening to my career? What will my future look like? Will I ever have time for myself again?"

Thirties Women stand on a solid footing. With new self-confidence and life experience, their connection to their spirituality is stronger than ever before in their lives. They can draw their boundaries to keep relationships in line. Rather than trying to distance themselves from their families as they did in their teens and twenties, Thirties Women appreciate the great value of a strong support system of extended family and friends, particularly if they have children of their own. As they begin to perceive that life is passing quickly, they feel an increasing urgency to live every day to the fullest.

WHAT THIRTIES WOMEN WORRY ABOUT

A woman who celebrates her thirty-first birthday today can expect to live at least another 51 years to become 82. Many will live much longer.

Although they have gained so much maturity and are beginning to feel— can you believe it? — like real adults, Thirties Women are still nearly as afraid of getting older as their Twenties sisters. The Thirties Women profiled here represent a wide range of attitudes and experiences. Lisa and Jennifer are afraid of getting older; Angela and Michelle are not. These women have more in common than not, yet still, each is unique. To be sure, none of them likes seeing her body change with the passing years, but the ones who are not afraid can accept these changes as inevitable. The fearful ones, in contrast, tend to fight aging with every fiber of their being.

Women fear to grow older for a variety of reasons. Where fewer than one-fifth of Twenties Women mentioned a concern for their health, more than a third of Thirties Women say health is their biggest aging concern. Increasingly targeted by cosmetic advertisements, Thirties Women also have become more concerned about their appearance. In this decade women feel very strong psychologically; where 13 percent of Twenties Women worried about their mental health, fewer than five percent of Thirties Women worry about it. Thirties Women stand tall and strong.

It's a great age, and many women say 30 or 35 is the age they most wished they could be. That's interesting, because women do not have a name for the years between 30 and 40; it's really a "no-woman's land." Women of all ages say "young" is under 30 and "middle-aged" starts around 40. But there's no name for the years in between 30 and 40. Thirties Women may wonder where they fit in this no-woman's land, but most are too busy to worry about it. Instead, they relish their unprecedented freedom to try out various paths as they chart their futures.

In this chapter we learn how Lisa, Angela, Jennifer, and Michelle gain confidence in their families and careers and assume adult roles in their communities. Strong, energetic, and ambitious, they have high expectations of themselves and may judge themselves and other women harshly. Although they may retain a strong circle of women friends from high school and college, their fears of appearing inadequate often keep them from sharing their true feelings with their peers.

LISA: "HAVING THE KIDS MAKES ME FEEL SO MUCH OLDER."

Lisa, 33, is so busy with kids and home and community that she meets herself coming and going. She married at age 28, determined to have her babies before she got too old. Now, life as a stay-at-home mom with two children under three takes all her time and energy.

Her husband is 19 years older and only 5 years younger than her parents; she has a stepson who is just 10 years younger than she. This fluidity of age confuses her and she was shocked when her female gynecologist commented that a third child, should she have one, would be coming "late in life."

Her husband travels all the time for work, so she has lots of parenting responsibility. "I am now realizing what a big job my mother had raising all of us as a single parent," says Lisa. "I thank her more each day, and am beginning to understand the great personal sacrifices she made to give us a nice home. Somehow she always made the time to be with us while we were growing up, which I realize now meant she had no other life outside of her work and us kids."

Lisa is so happy now, that her only wish is that she could have a little more quiet "me" time now rather than later, when she grows older. "I'm afraid then I will be so lonely without my children," she says.

"I know I am at one of the best ages yet," she acknowledges. She is smart, pretty, has a wonderfully supportive husband, and beautiful, healthy children. So what's wrong? She can't stop thinking about the passage of time and she is afraid of growing older. "What is creepy is I know that time is running out and I am beginning to see changes in my skin and hair, and my energy levels have dropped, and I am fighting added pounds that do not want to come off."

She wishes she could stop aging and worries about wrinkles and staying young looking. "Having the kids makes me feel so much older and, of course, more responsible. I have to think about the future for my children's sake and I have to be healthy and strong for them."

Although her husband tries to reassure her, deep down Lisa feels afraid she won't be desirable any more. This creates problems in their relationship that bewilder him. She wonders, "Will I be able to keep my wonderful mate? Will he still love me even if I'm not as cute and sexy as I once was? What if he meets someone out of town?

"I'm afraid that men won't do things for me as they did when I was young," she says. "When I was younger I didn't think much about getting older. Now I am older and wiser and know a lot more of the things that can happen later in life."

Her relationship needs have changed from her twenties only in that her circle of friends now needs to include people who understand family-related pressures. "We need relationships with couples who are like us and our families." Although she still dearly loves her remaining single friends, their lives are so very different that sometimes it's hard to find things in common beyond their shared past. "Another challenge is that many of my girlfriends are working moms," she says, "and I feel like they look down on me for staying home, although they deny it." She worries that she is not as interesting as her friends now that her job involves catering to toddlers 24/7.

She hasn't worked since her second child was born. Truth be known, the women in their fifties and sixties who had been there a long time drove her out of her last job. They undermined her and made her life miserable. "I wasn't the first they had run off.

"Ultimately they asked me to leave saying 'You just don't fit in,' but it was actually for the best because I was able to get unemployment and stay home with the kids." She found great solace and support from other members of her professional association, who helped her get over her pain and fury.

Although she mostly enjoys her stay-at-home status, it is only temporary. When her little one goes to school, their financial plan requires her to return to the workplace, and she will once again call on her mentors to help guide her reentry into the workforce.

Lisa focuses on improving both her physique and her emotional well-being by trying to maintain a youthful appearance. "I use a lot of skin care products, and keep waiting for them to deliver on the promises of making me lose 10 years in seven days," Lisa says. "Not to mention the pills that were supposed to bust the fat right off my body."

She resolved part of her worry about her appearance by getting a breast lift and augmentation after she stopped nursing her second baby. "I always had a really cute bust line and I was not about to let that go," she says.

Keeping her exercise plan afloat is a constant challenge with the two kids, but she knows she *must* remain physically fit. It's the only way she will have the energy and motivation to care for their family and herself. It's also essential to keeping her depression under control. The more exercise, the fewer antidepressants she needs.

Lisa really hates to think about getting older, and avoids it if she can. "Aging to me means all the things I will not be able to do and how my health will be when I'm older," says Lisa. "I don't want my children to have to take care of me." Lisa's mother worships beauty and youth, and that has affected how she feels about aging. "She doesn't talk about this attitude," she says, "but I know that it affects her because she always tries to look younger.

"I hope my feelings are very different from hers," Lisa says, yet she has to admit she shares many of her mom's views. "I try to believe that women become more valuable as they age, but my mom believes the opposite."

Lisa's mother was widowed in her thirties, and she raised Lisa and her younger brother by working as a teacher. Lisa feels guilty about her mom's sacrifices and is sad that her mom seems to have given up. "My mother is a beautiful woman at age 58 but says that her time for finding another man is past. She thinks she's too old and dried up. So she keeps busy with her work and occupies her time with her friends and hobbies. But I would want more. I want to feel young and not ever feel that time is passing me by. If anything happened to my husband, no way I could stay alone. I would want to marry again."

To keep their lifestyle going on her husband's income alone, Lisa has to plan well and spend wisely. She's lucky to live near extended family members, who provide love, support, and childcare so she and her husband can go out on an occasional date. She tries to return the favor.

"I try to show my older family members all the love and compassion that I can," she says. "Even when they make outrageous requests, I try to fulfill them. Life is short, and once that person is gone I don't want that guilty feeling that I wish I had spent more time with them.

· ·

I am not living the same life my parents and grandparents did, so I should not compare myself to them.

· ·

"I feel good about myself when I am involved in something at church or my kids' school," says Lisa. "It's important to me to do a good job at something. I like working hard in my garden and in my house. We are all uniquely beautiful and wonderfully made in the image of God. I tell my girlfriends that I call my SUV my chapel. While I drive so often I'm praying, "Please God, help me be a patient, understanding mother. Help me not be scared. Help me remember that I don't have to make sense of it, just accept it."

When she's feeling strong, Lisa knows each woman needs to discover her own gifts and talents and put them to use. She believes we are here for a reason, and that God always has a plan. "I hope I make the right choice in all areas now," says Lisa, "for my finances, my health, and my heart."

. . . .

LISA IS A VERY BUSY Thirties Woman. She is always multi-tasking with her family and volunteer work. Among her many strengths are her spirituality, her ties to her friends and family, and her church. She is hard-working, with a lot of skills. As delighted as she is with her status in a clearly adult world, she judges herself harshly and struggles with self-doubt. This is one of her greatest challenges.

Stay-at-home moms like Lisa worry that their friends might find them boring, or feel defensive about leaving the workforce. The truth is, although their friends may periodically stir up competition, rivalry, and criticism of each other, these days they're too busy thinking about their own problems. If Thirties Women can let go of this self-conscious worry, they can restore the closeness they crave.

Keeping energy and motivation high so they can care for their families — and themselves — drives these women's health and exercise plans. Lisa feels conflicted about her mother; although she is grateful, she does not want to end up like her Mom. Without a positive role model, women like Lisa dread the thought of giving up a lost youth. This fear is driven strongly by the advertising message, "If you want to be loved you must stay, young and beautiful," seen everywhere on magazines and billboards that display young, impossibly thin, and gorgeous women. A lot of Thirties Women are talking about where to get the latest and greatest beauty treatments, and Lisa is listening like she never did before. "Some of my friends are getting on the Beauty Boat," she says, "and I wonder sometimes if I'll miss the ship."

As far as we're concerned, if a breast procedure makes a woman feel more confident, why not? Even though Lisa feels some of her girlfriends criticize her for worrying about her appearance, that is her right. We are each different and should just paddle our own boats and never mind. No one has the right to judge another.

Women like Lisa can overcome their fears by expressing them to other women her own age. They need to know that they are not alone and that many other women share the fear that they will become "invisible" when their beauty fades. When a woman's personal value depends on her physical appearance, she will naturally feel fearful and anxious about her future.

Lisa needs support now to dispel her distorted thoughts about her future. Female mentors are available if women will look for them. Although a stay-at-home mom may not want to enter the job market now there are many ways to stay current. She can reconnect and keep active in a professional organization; take courses to remain marketable and up to date; or work part time for a social-profit organization. Volunteering to help these organizations can build confidence and show women they still have the talents and skills that are needed in the working world.

All of these things will keep her in the know about her ever-changing field of interest. This will help to build her self-confidence and stop some of the negative, destructive thoughts she is having. If she feels she needs more help, I encourage her to meet with a professional about her concerns and talk out some of her fears.

ANGELA: "FRIENDSHIPS HAVE BECOME SO MUCH MORE IMPORTANT TO ME."

Angela, 37, works full time to support her three children. She divorced five years ago, isn't a bit afraid of getting older, and loves to sing, laugh, and have a good time. Her friends love her energy and sparkle.

She feels healthy mentally and knows what is important to her, even though her twenties were difficult. "My kids have been great, and they have made me less self-centered because I focus on them," she says. One challenge has been balancing the needs of her kids and family members in town, and developing relationships with friends who have children. They do play dates, but the married moms don't invite her to couples parties.

"Friendships have become so much more important to me. Friends are my outlet, my stability. But I have enjoyed growing older, and have gotten clarity on which ones are my lifelong friends, not just people to party with, but someone to relate when a child is up sick all night. We can do it together."

Even so, she contemplates her upcoming twentieth high school reunion with utter disbelief. "I think about aging quite often, at least several times a week," Angela says, "but it doesn't scare me." She teaches dance and can feel her body beginning to rebel with knee and back problems. The worst part of getting older, she fears, will be a loss of her ability to move and enjoy the wonderful sights, smells, sounds, touch, and tastes of this amazing world.

"I work with people who were born as I was getting out of high school. That can be a bit difficult, because at times I feel no older than my students. I have a 16-year-old daughter, which confuses me because I still feel that age myself. It's weird. I have a hard time adjusting to that."

Right now Angela is in a relationship with a man four years older than herself, which makes her think of the passing years more often than if she were with someone closer to her own age. He doesn't have much interest in her kids, which makes her wonder if she'll ever find a mate to help raise her family.

Although she would really like to re-marry, her boyfriend, who has grown kids of his own, shows no interest in that. She loves him but knows he does not offer the future she wants. Because she spends almost all her time either working or taking care of her kids, she wonders how she could ever meet a different man.

Single parenthood is so difficult that she would like to find someone with the same goals and ambitions for a stable family with whom she could share the rest of her life. In the wee hours after a difficult day, she yearns to have someone to depend on, someone willing to make a commitment. Fortunately, she has plenty of divorced friends with kids who help support and encourage each other.

"I never thought I would be worried about measuring up to other women," she says, "but so many men seem to be interested only in younger women." Much as she rejects society's focus on youth and beauty, she still sometimes wonders, "Am I still attractive? Am I hitting a middle-age crisis?

"On the plus side, I do like the wisdom that I have gained and the experiences that make me who I am," she says. "I can't wait for more!" Angela nurtures herself with meditation, engaging in outdoor adventures, and being friendly and open-minded to other people. "I'm continually seeking knowledge and trying to become a better person," she says.

Her friends consider her something of a maverick. "I don't want to be forced into conformity, to be behaviorally modified through rewards and punishments such that I limit my freedom to think independently," she says. "I don't want to get set in my ways, and I really don't want to lose my hope and ability to dream of future possibilities.

"I've always tried to have control over my health and do the things I can, like eating well and exercising," says Angela. "It is very important for me to always have something that is just for me, like marathon training or volunteering."

She places less emphasis on her looks per se than on her physical performance as a runner. "I have always loved to run. One of the biggest wake-ups for me was while training for a marathon. I had a calf injury, the first injury that ever really held me back. I read that calf strains mostly happen to people over 30. Hello, that's me.

"What a great lesson. I focused on stretching, icing, and heat application to make myself feel better. I also accepted in my heart and soul that I might not complete the marathon. I would have been disappointed but I knew I had done everything I could to make it better. That is the attitude I want to adopt as I grow older: to do the best I can to nurture my body while accepting whatever is. As it turns out, I completed the marathon feeling strong and steady." She's also making the best of the news that another knee problem stems from early arthritis.

Angela struggles to keep from buying into the youth-and-beauty culture. "Women need to be valued for being people, not objects. It ties in to what you work out for yourself. What do you really value? How do you perceive yourself? We all start out perceiving ourselves through the eyes of others, but as we mature, we get over that to develop our own sense of self.

"However, I am starting to notice that I look tired in the morning. I see my wrinkles and wonder what I will look like in the future. It is very hard to have a flat stomach like I did when I was younger but I feel stronger than ever, too. I hope that I can look like a distinguished older person, rather than just someone old trying to look young.

"I think I worry mostly about gaining weight and not being able to lose it," Angela says. "I have never been skinny and have always had to work on it. I know it is going to get harder and I just want to look the best I can."

....

I am comfortable and happy with myself and I do not need other people's approval.

....

Angela's mother has struggled with her aging appearance and recently had a facelift. "I did not think she needed it but I respected that she was doing what she needed to do for herself. Actually, the surgery seems to have given her more confidence and she is enjoying herself more. It's a barrier between us in a way — we have never talked about it."

In her darkest moments Angela worries about "not being able to support myself, about providing for my children's future, and ending up alone. What kind of life will I have in 25 years? How will I have changed or grown? What will I have accomplished? I hope I'm not wasting any precious time then wondering if I'm doing the right thing or not."

To counteract her anxiety about the future, Angela saves money in a plan at work. "I know it is not much but I hope to do more. Many of my friends have not considered saving yet." She wants to be fully in charge of her future, and it bothers her that she doesn't have the money to pursue more education or job training right now. She's determined to get there soon, however, because she hates the prospect of forever worrying about money and health care and her children's futures. She wants to buy a home and a better car and is trying to become better off financially now, while she can do more things with her children. She says, "Part of taking care of myself means earning a decent living, planning well, and spending wisely."

She admires her sister, who went to medical school and now juggles a busy practice and three kids, but she can't imagine having that kind of drive herself. "My sister believes she is a better mother when she uses her God-given skills to help others. She works hard all day as a physician, but when she gets home, she is eager to hug and kiss them and be the best mother she can be. "I don't understand how she does it, but my sister can't *not* do it. She thinks her children will someday appreciate having a mother who is trying to make a difference in the world, and instead of feeling guilty, she feels determined." Although Angela daydreams about feeling called to a career, she hasn't heard it yet.

Lacking a spouse, Angela has built a support network, feels the respect of her peers, and cherishes her mentors. "My great aunts are 82 and 86," Angela says. "They still drive, live on their own, and one of them still wears kicky skirts and go-go boots! They are excellent role models, absolutely beautiful people and I don't mean physical appearance. They are extraordinary on the inside, always helping others. I admire that."

When Angela feels down, her morning pep talks to herself are variations on a theme: "Stand up straight and stand up for your beliefs. I'm doing the best I can. Nothing is forever. The only constant is change, and I put forth the effort to bring about change. I am so blessed. God, please give me the wisdom to live each day to its fullest. Age is a state of mind, and I am just me. I believe in myself. I am only as old as I feel."

If I can continue to believe in myself, I am only as old as I feel.

Most of the time, Angela is serenely happy. "I really like this age because I spend less time worrying about what other people think of me," she says. "Instead, I'm finding people I feel comfortable with and who feel the same way with me."

. . . .

ANGELA HAS STRENGTHS THAT HELP her meet life's challenges. She has humor, laughter, sparkle, and a strong faith. She draws people to her with her energy and works to keep herself healthy by maintaining her commitment to exercise and taking responsibility for herself. She is practical yet hopeful, and consciously uses positive self-talk to keep herself on track emotionally. And she understands the importance of her deep values and she is not afraid of getting older.

Like other women blindsided by divorce, her challenges center on her finances. At 35, she is already finding it harder to teach dance, which is a tremendously athletic discipline. With her leg injuries and arthritis in her knee, she faces the same dilemma as a ballplayer. Although athletes with tremendous discipline can perform into their forties, most are happier if they find an alternative career before then.

Angela's greatest fear is that she will get sick and be unable to work. Thirties Women often find their first serious injury or health problem brings them important lessons in maturity and self-care. Angela hasn't seen it yet, but this was a wake-up call for her career. She needs to go to her area community college or university and have a serious talk with the guidance and financial aid counselors to explore her interests, abilities, and prospects. She can also draw upon her strong network of friends and family. Tackling a big goal like a career change is like eating an elephant. You can only do it one bite at a time.

Angela is one of the many single mothers in the United States working hard to take care of herself and her three children. They do not have time to think about much beyond their basic needs, but they need to carve out the time to plan for themselves. As their children grow older, they will be able to take more time for themselves that they can devote to developing more profitable careers.

Support systems are more important than ever for these women and they need to accept all the help they can get. Angela has been fortunate. She had the advantage of watching and interacting with women in her family and has seen many examples of positive aging. Although her priorities are different, Angela accepts and honors people like her mother who focuses on her appearance. Each woman has to choose for herself what she believes is important. A great many women like Angela have never really adopted the beauty culture and instead prefer to accept their lives and enjoy each day.

Thirties Women can be wonderful mentors for other women of any age. Everyone benefits from talking with other women who have been down the same path. Women are too often caught completely unprepared by divorce or the death of a spouse, and experienced mentors can help them consider their financial value and security.

At this stage, Angela might consider a life coach to help her to review what she wants. Although she might wish she could be a stay-at-home mom that seems an unlikely prospect at this point. When a woman finds out what really makes her happy she can develop a plan for herself. Should Angela open her own dance studio? Or should she move into an entirely new career that would allow her to work at home, spend time with the kids and, still "pump up the volume" on her earnings and life satisfaction.

Angela has great things going for herself. Divorce is just a blip on the screen. She has the great opportunity now to pilot her own ship, lead her own army, direct her own life, and fill it with purpose and passion. When women cultivate their own interests and passions, life becomes more exciting and their life prospects do improve.

JENNIFER: "WILL I EVER MARRY?"

Jennifer, age 35, feels coolly confident and quite pleased with her life. After completing her graduate degree, Jennifer immediately landed her dream job and is now making good money as a financial advisor. "I am so excited to at last be capable of caring for myself and not having to worry so much about my future," she says. "By now, I have co-workers who appreciate me for my intelligence and *what* I know, rather than for what I look like, or *who* I know."

It wasn't always this way. At first, Jennifer had to prove herself, not just because she was a woman, but also because she was young. A lot of the other employees were men, 40 to 60 years old. "It was probably easier for me than for some women," she says, "because I was 'raised by wolves.'" Growing up in a family of boys, Jennifer learned to be strong and independent and to relate comfortably with men. They taught me it wasn't about my looks. I realized women worry the most about their appearance mostly for what other *women* think of them. Men don't really notice that much.

The models in women's magazines are airbrushed, not perfect!

"Still it was a struggle to hold my own and compete. I always wore very conservative pants, vests, and jackets to work because I didn't want the wrong kind of attention from the men."

No matter what the future brings, Jennifer wants to be able to take care of herself. "I see friends really struggling to pay their bills and for their health care, and I know how important it is for women to plan for their futures. I believe that a woman should be independent and not totally rely on her mate," says Jennifer. "We have to look to ourselves (not to a man or any other person) for our own happiness and love ourselves no matter what. No matter who else is in your life, you have to take care of yourself first; don't worry about what others think of you. It ties in to what you work out for yourself."

Although she has had much career success, she feels unsatisfied on some level and judges herself harshly, saying, "I wish that I would have done more with my life up to this point and had more to show for my years. Someday, though, I hope to finally get it through my thick skull that I am one neat lady, no matter how much I weigh or how many wrinkles I develop! I think of aging more now that I am no longer the youngest everywhere I go."

Jennifer is an independent thinker when it comes to relationships. Having seen older women put up with lousy relationships because they could not earn their own living, she is fiercely determined to make her own way. "I am not married and really not sure if I will find Mr. Right, and even if I did, he could easily morph into Mr. Wrong."

She always assumed her thirties would bring her love and the family she longs for. "I just felt like it would happen when I was ready. Many of my friends have married recently and I am becoming the lone single one. I am getting tried of being the bridesmaid waiting for that throwing-the-bouquet moment. I am torn between catching the darn thing or just stepping aside for the panting, excited woman pressing against my back."

Sometimes she feels guilty that she enjoys a freedom that others do not because she doesn't have kids yet. "But people always ask: 'Why aren't you married?' And it's awful when people ask me about having children. It makes me want to cram it down their throats. Don't they realize how that makes me feel? Living in a conservative part of the country, it seems that is an expectation. But I like what I do and wonder, 'Why can't I have it all?' "

I remind myself that millions of other people are in the same boat as me.

Aging parents and a career are her main priorities, and she struggles with relationship issues. She likes to work really hard — a lot — and her boyfriends haven't really understood that about her.

Jennifer is afraid of getting older. When she wakes in the night she wonders, "Will I ever marry? Will I ever find someone with the same priorities for their work, family, and personal life? Will I be able to afford decent living conditions? Who will take care of me? Will I have regrets for not doing certain things or taking chances?"

Jennifer wants a family of her own — just not quite yet — and it weighs on her mind. "I am always worrying that I won't be able to have the large family that I want, because I am getting too old. When will be the appropriate time to have a child? I am not ready yet. However, everyone else seems to have an opinion about it. I have faith that advances in science, technology, and medicine allow for women like me to accomplish career goals before embarking on the child-rearing stage. I also feel healthy. However, people warn me, 'Do not wait too long.' What is 'too long'?"

Hanging around her married friends who have children really reminds Jennifer of aging. So does helping her father take care of her aging grandparents, although mostly that reminds her to enjoy every single day. In truth, she is so busy she has little time to fret. Right now she is focused on buying her second home and a new car. Then she wants to get back to traveling. "I'm doing well, I think, but I often wonder how I compare to others in my financial preparations. Will I be OK?"

Jennifer feels torn. She wants to be a good daughter, granddaughter, career woman, and girlfriend and sometimes wonders if she is doing any of it well. Her commitment to helping her father and grandparents adds a layer of complication to her search for both a committed relationship and career advancement. "I love my job and have worked hard to get to this level. But they want me to travel now and my Dad's health is iffy and Gram and Gramps need more and more help. I know I could hire someone to help them, but I am not so sure I trust anyone."

Her boyfriend broke up with her because she didn't have enough time for him, and he was tired of waiting around. She knows something has to change, but doesn't know what that might be. All these demands make it a challenge to keep a relationship, and seeing her boyfriend's commitment fade leaves her feeling insecure.

Jennifer has noticed that she is no longer so interested in being the life of the party and dancing until the sun comes up. "I just don't have the energy. I think more about getting my eight hours of sleep so I can stay on top of my game and get that promotion! I watch the younger men and women partying on and think, "Yikes! That was me 10 years ago!"

Her greatest worry is that she might get sick. As a single person, Jennifer does not have a built-in support system. There is no spouse to count on. The worst part about getting older, she thinks, would be losing the ability to be active with your kids and partner. Feeling the years march by, she wishes she had her previous energy level back, and that her metabolism would kick back in.

Jennifer misses her mom, who died of cancer at age 47 when Jennifer was a teenager. Because they were close, she dreams of having a daughter of her own and seeing her become a woman. However, she realizes that losing her mother at such an early age has left her with little information about what life will be like as she grows older. She says, "I try not to think about cancer but catch myself wondering if I will die like my mother did at 47. I do have an older cousin who is healthy, though. She seems happy and, in her sixties, she's full of adventure and her new boyfriend has given her a new outlook on love and life."

"I will always try to stay stylish and fit, but it is creepy to watch television and see how all these women use surgery to keep themselves looking young and beautiful," Jennifer says. "What is more important to my self-image is knowing who I am and what is going on around me."

Jennifer says, "I look at older women and think 'that will be me sometime soon'!" Through her church she has found a group of women of all ages with whom she is able to share some her thoughts about aging. "They are helping me look in the mirror now and just see what a nice person I am."

....

JENNIFER WONDERS WHAT SHE WILL have to give up in order to achieve her goals of balancing career with family. Thirties Women who are single want love, understanding, and their own income security, although they may wonder if those goals can coexist or if they are harboring a fantasy. Although Jennifer has had several relationships over time, none has stuck. Sometimes it makes her nervous how comfortable she has become with her single life. When she realistically takes stock of her goals and the nature of her relationships so far, she has begun to consider the possibility that she may never marry.

Women who face this possibility take stock of their strengths. Their self-sufficiency and strong earning ability make it possible for them to consider building a satisfying life without Prince Charming. For Thirties Women, being able to finally take care of themselves signifies a real developmental passage. It marks their transition from dependency to a bright future of personal security, and they see themselves as confident, capable, and healthy humans.

A Thirties Woman who has never married may worry about missing out on children and having no one to spend the rest of her life with. Being without a mate does not necessarily mean a woman has to go it alone, though, and she can build wonderful support networks among friends, professional contacts, and church. Such a network will literally be a lifesaver both in caring for her and for her aging family members.

Just being asked about their aging process helps Thirties Women see more clearly how they fit into the world. They are surprised — and relieved — to find they are not alone in wondering about growing older and what they will be like as older women. It enrages single women that perfect strangers will nose into their plans for marriage and children, but this is human nature. Because Jennifer is so successful, people want to comment on the area where she is not successful. She needs to learn to laugh at this and not let it bother her.

As for having children, adoption is a popular option for single women. Jennifer's friend Connor gave up on finding a "perfect man" and opted instead for the "perfect sperm donor." At first Connor's parents were shocked, but then decided they *really* wanted grandchildren, so why not? Their grandson is now a year old and mom and grandparents are all thrilled.

Women are waiting longer than ever to begin their reproductive lives because they expect technology to let them become mothers at any time. The technologies they count on to extend their chances of later-life pregnancy include fertility drugs, freezing eggs, and donor eggs. Women who want to bear a child themselves may be surprised to learn that some women can enter perimenopause — the beginning of the end of their fertile cycles — before they even leave their twenties. Of course, a surrogate mother also may be a viable option.

Although Jennifer is aware of her many options, she also realizes children (and subsequent grandchildren) may never happen. She comforts herself with the knowledge that there are a lot of married people who should not have kids and who should not even be married. Even without children of their own, Thirties Women may begin the sandwich generation experience of caring for aging family members. This is a stressful and demanding time when a woman's personal needs for time and space typically take a back seat to the needs of others.

MICHELLE: "WE HAVE SURVIVED THE JUGGLING MATCH!"

Michelle, 39, got married in her early twenties. Her children have now nearly completed high school. Her issue today is balancing her family and career with her need for at least a little time for herself. "It's hard when working full time," she says. "I feel like I am judged for working rather than staying home, but I don't care. Work is my 'me-time.'"

"We have survived the juggling match!" Michelle says excitedly. Married for nearly 20 years, she and her high school sweetheart have weathered many changes in their relationship: his work, her work, attraction to others, tough travel schedules, sick kids, worries, exhaustion, no time for romance … and they have come to accept and appreciate each other for who they are. "After all the work of raising our family, my husband and I are looking forward to more freedom and adventure. He was so supportive, and always made sure I got some time away from the stresses of motherhood."

She has found such joy in her secure marriage. "I hope that my husband and I live a full, happy, healthy life, still in love, clear of mind, able to take care of ourselves into old age, and that we have many grandchildren and great-grandchildren." Although family occupies much of her mind, her aging concerns center more on her work life. "It's a bit scary to think about where my career will go because I've still got 20 or 30 more years of work left in me."

Michelle struggled with societal expectations and her sense of somehow falling short. "When I was turning 30 I felt like I had to really produce something in my life. I had tried so many things and now I personally felt it was time to make up my mind and find the "right path." I have started my own design company and it is scary but I am really excited about producing something that I can be proud of." Starting her own company helped Michelle feel like at last she is fulfilling her potential.

Like many working moms, Michelle has continued to work her whole life, except for taking the minimum pregnancy leave with each of her kids. And like most working moms, she wishes she had more help at home. Michelle rarely thinks about her looks, perhaps partly because she is so busy. She says, "I rarely have time to look in the mirror, much less worry about getting older. All I want is to have the energy to keep up with my business and my busy family.

"Getting older is something to look forward to. The alternative to aging is being dead. Your age is just a number. It's your state of mind that's important. If you are comfortable with yourself everything else will just fall into place.

"I do worry that things will happen to my family. I'm scared for my friends, too, so it's probably denial that I don't really worry about me. However, after watching my sister-in-law die of cancer at age 42, I know for a fact that life is much too short. My sister-in-law taught me to look forward to birthdays because that's another year God has given the gift of sharing your life with your loved ones." Having witnessed this untimely death, she is not really afraid of getting older.

Maturing has its advantages. "I think I get better looking the older I get, and I am very excited about how much more I understand about myself as time goes by," she says. "I'm much more comfortable in my own skin. I know now that with age comes greater wisdom, and I surely know a heck of a lot more now than I did 10 years ago." If Michelle has any fear at all, it is of not living now, while she has the chance.

Thirties Women want to enjoy life to the fullest. "I want to enjoy my youth while it lasts so I'll be happily burned out when I'm older," says Michelle. "I want to keep doing what I'm used to doing, traveling, loving my husband, and going out and having a good time, all the things I like to do. I am going to turn 40 soon and I want to do like my grandmother and 'burn out, not rust out.' I want to live life to the fullest and not have any regrets about what I never got to do. I do not want to be afraid of anything.

"Getting older is easier to accept when we can joke and share stories of our experiences," she says. Her stress management program involves "surrounding myself with good, fun people and taking mini-vacations to unwind, even if it is just for an afternoon."

Even though she accepts it as inevitable, she thinks of aging every day. "I realize I can't look the way I did 10 years ago and I struggle with accepting that maybe I won't ever lose that five pounds," she says. "But I sure will keep trying — while also balancing that goal with eating my favorite things like chocolate chip cookies!"

Michelle rarely sinks into an aging funk, but when she does, Alzheimer's dominates her thoughts. Several family members have developed the disease, one at the young age of 65. "My biggest fear is losing my mind," she says. "That scares me to death." That actually scares her much more than dying. "I got over my fear of death by getting really close to it myself," she says. "We should feel special and lucky that we are able to experience aging, because so many of us women die young."

Michelle's mother has taken growing older in stride. "At age 69 her attitude is 'Take what comes your way and make the best of it.' She has never colored her hair, now salt-and-pepper, nor made any surgical changes, and she wears little makeup. It's not because she doesn't care, because she looks great," Michelle says. "She is sensible, healthy, works out, and takes care of herself. She truly has taken whatever has come her way (including an extra unwanted 30 pounds), accepted it, and made the best of it.

Michelle says, "I think she has aged beautifully. She also has never really talked about 'getting older.' She just leads by example. Her parents died recently, and, as the eldest of nine children, she has taken on the role of matriarch of the family. So getting older for her has meant becoming the head of the family and taking over where her parents left off.

Some Thirties Women perceive that society doesn't value its older members enough. But Michelle doesn't see such discrimination. "People appreciate you for your intelligence and what you have learned," she says, "Not for what you look like, or who you know. Nonetheless, feeling part of a community helps a lot, as does enjoying time with my friends and earning respect from my peers.

. . . .

You can't turn back the clock,
but you can wind it up again.

. . . .

"My grandmother also never ceases to amaze me with her energy and zest for life," says Michelle. "She travels to far-away places and is open to new and exciting things. I think she stays young in heart and spirit and that is what makes her so much fun to be around. She also never judges anyone and has a nice word and quick smile for all she meets."

Michelle views the changes in her physical appearance as battle scars. "I can accept myself as I am, with a little help from make-up, hair coloring, and staying physically fit. My biggest problem really is finding clothes that fit my personality and shape. It's funny how challenging that is. I am fit and am always mistaken for a younger person, but I want nice, age-appropriate clothes — not things my 16-year-old would wear. There's a lack of this sort of clothing. When I get older I want to be one of those cute, snappy-dressing, make-up-wearing active little ladies that play bingo and go to senior citizen dances."

One unsettling fact: her hormones have started fluctuating, and she thinks she's starting perimenopause, although everyone assures her she is much too young. "Aging is a fact of life," Michelle says. "Being in my thirties has uplifted my sense of comfort within my skin and spiritual resistance to outside forces that try to intervene. I just try to do my best and remember that not everyone can be a super mom, tireless worker, or perfect wife."

For those who have successfully weathered the storms and built a happy, stable marriage, getting older together is a wonderfully comforting and attractive prospect. "I think about retirement and traveling with my husband in an RV around the country," says Michelle. "I enjoy life and the way my husband looks at me makes me feel really good about myself.

"Knowing my children will be there for me, having grandchildren, and being able to do things I can't now," are the things Michelle most looks forward to about growing older. "Also, I think about the rich life and many accomplishments the elderly people I know have achieved in their lifetime, and hope I will have done the same."

After she completes her remaining decades of work life, Michelle looks forward to the metaphorical fall of her life, when she will sit back, watch the leaves turn colors, and put the insecurities and pressures of youth behind her. "It will be wonderful not to have to rush around all the time," she says. "With maturity and experience I expect to be able to see how far I have come and not feel out of place. I think that the way you feel about yourself inside is what you will show to others. If I feel good about myself, other people will see my wise side. Surely aging is about learning and getting better. As long as I can feel good about that, everything else works out just fine."

For Michelle, her faith has become a vital comfort and support. Michelle says, "My sister-in-law was a dear friend and I could not believe I would lose her so soon. After she died I started going to church again and have joined the young married group. I feel at peace and I treasure my spiritual connection."

. . . .

BECAUSE SHE ACCEPTS THAT AGING will happen, Michelle is able to reframe it into a positive force in her life. She talks comfortably about aging, even about death, with her friends. Her other strengths include a strong faith, an extended traditional family network, and realistic expectations about what she will be able to accomplish. Her successful marriage is a rock her entire family leans on.

One of her major challenges is running and increasing her own design business. As an entrepreneur, she is finding the demands much greater than she had expected, and her children are complaining. Another challenge is that her husband has always taken care of the finances, in their marriage and in her business. Sure, she had her hands full, and after all, he is an accountant — but still. Michelle is woefully unprepared to handle her own finances should anything happen to her husband.

The tension between having children and keeping their careers going is a continual pull on the two-thirds of mothers who work outside the home. Their major concerns include finding help with the children and homes and raising their children in a safe and emotionally stable environment.

....

I look forward to aging, for with it comes wisdom, freedom, strength. There is so much to look forward to, and I am not afraid to show my age.

....

Women like Michelle have a balanced view. They have worked to fulfill the dreams of their twenties. As is often the case when a woman does well with aging, Michelle's mother has been a wonderful role model, even though she does not talk with her daughter about it. When they are fortunate enough to be close to their mothers, both emotionally and geographically, Thirties Women can gain a pretty clear picture of what to expect. However, if the mother keeps her internal feelings secret, this is a shame, because talking about their feelings can help Thirties Women avoid guilt and confusion when their turn as matriarch comes.

Seeing a mother step into the role of family matriarch helps Thirties Women see that life is cyclical. They can be comfortable with having aging parents to care for as well as school-age children and they expect this pattern to play out in their own lifetimes. When they can no longer care for themselves, they trust that other family members will step into the caregiver role.

Women is this age group are already trying on ideas of what kind of older woman they want to be: quietly joyful, bitter and complaining, full of fun, eccentric, unconventional, or old and burned out? Michelle also has several older friends who have invented their own version of "getting old." She says, "They are constantly going off to some far-away place, river rafting, hiking up mountains, and wearing whatever they want. I want to be like that, no one to tell me what to do or what to wear or what to be."

Coming to some kind of peace is a helpful strategy for many busy women and they also want to share with their own children the importance of being more accepting of themselves. A faithful and nurturing relationship with a spouse or a companion leads to healthy and happy experiences for women in their thirties and beyond.

The most common themes, for Michelle, focus on things that are central to her being: self-assurance and not caring about what others think, having a good sense of herself, being comfortable and happy with herself, and not needing the approval of others. Women like Michelle know it's best to accept that aging is natural and that there is no way to avoid it.

WHAT DO THIRTIES WOMEN WANT?

Thirties Women have weathered the insecurities of the twenties to encounter greater confidence and security. In doing so, they enter a no-man's land. They are no longer really young, yet they are clearly not yet middle-aged. My research showed women actually have no name to identify this period of their lives.

The Thirties are a poignant time, when women gain an understanding of consequences much deeper than in the twenties. They are incredibly busy, with their lives spinning full speed ahead. Facing daily choices has made them realize it is not possible to walk all paths and pursue all opportunities in a single lifetime.

Ultimately each Thirties Woman must strike her own balance. Each has a different set of challenges and realities for her health, financial stability, relationships, and issues surrounding her aging process.

THE PICTURE OF HEALTH

Thirties Women are a lot more together psychologically than their Twenties sisters. Lisa uses exercise and antidepressants to control her depression. Although they have taken on more responsibilities in their thirties, they're not much more worried about money and being alone than the Twenties. There is one area in which they are noticeably more worried, in fact, twice as worried. Like Angela who worked for months to recover from a calf injury, they are paying a lot more attention to their health.

Compared to Twenties Women, still insulated by the perceived invulnerability of youth, Thirties Women get a dose of physical reality. Their bodies have begun to change; they see serious illness in family members and friends — even themselves. Fortunately, education appears to be making an impact on younger women, who are becoming more aware of heart disease and other diseases that affect women. The rising cost of health care is on every woman's mind.

Even so, as "Dr. Mom," the Thirties Woman tends to focus her worrying on other people: parents, kids, spouse, and co-workers. Her own healthcare needs stay unnoticed on the back burner until some kind of crisis becomes a major health concern. Most don't yet struggle with common issues like high blood pressure, although Michelle's hormones are waning and Jennifer has arthritis.

Such physical changes can erode self-esteem and they must draw upon their increasing self-confidence to steady themselves. But all Thirties Women, fearful or not, are awakening to health issues. In these reproductive years, gynecological worries take the lead, as does staying healthy for kids and jobs. The dramatic loss of friends and family members to cancer often gives them a false impression of their true lifetime risk, so they don't yet think of threats like heart disease.

It's vitally important that Thirties Women talk with their doctors to assess their true risk of the various diseases that kill women, including heart disease, cancer, lung diseases, and diabetes. Many of these have genetic components, and it's especially important to begin a program of early screening for women with a family history indicating increased risk.

Lisa and Jennifer are afraid of getting older and they are not alone. More than half of Thirties Women share their fear. They worry more than their fearless sisters about declining energy levels and health issues, including childbearing. Women who are afraid of aging are less confident that they will be able to care for themselves as they grow older.

In general, fearless women like Angela and Michelle ignore the downside of aging. They work to develop their careers, improve their finances and their quality of life, and pursue vibrant health. Rather than worrying about the loss of their youth, they perceive mature women as being happier and more interesting than younger women.

Angela and Michelle are taking aging in stride. They regard their added pounds and graying hair as just part of the natural process. Fortunate to have found good role models in either their mothers or another older person, they have chosen a positive road map to follow. If Mom is doing OK with the aging thing, her daughter is more likely to take it in stride as well. If Mom sees getting older as the end of everything good, her daughter often struggles as well. We learn best by example, and a positive role model can reassure and encourage us about what lies ahead.

. . . .

There are three billion women in the world
who don't look like super models
and only eight who do.

. . . .

To the extent that women worry about their health, they often focus on their weight. Women in the United States have been getting heavier in recent years, despite the massive diet industry. One conclusion is obvious: Diets don't work. Only when women can find for themselves a new relationship with food that focuses on their health rather than on the numbers on a scale, will they have a chance to move gradually toward a healthy weight.

DIETS DON'T WORK

Most people stay on them only a few days or months, and weight usually rebounds as soon as former patterns of eating and exercise are restored. The only way to slim down and keep weight off is to permanently change eating habits and increase levels of exercise, including both weight training and cardio exercises.

Learn about proper nutrition and teach the family so that children will learn to eat healthy too. To identify emotional or impulse eating, write down all foods eaten, note when and where they were eaten and any emotions experienced at the time. Stress levels affect food consumption and can cause other health issues, so it's useful for a woman to chart her stress level on a scale of 1 (high stress) to 10 (low stress).

A woman needs to be kind to herself. Healthy eating and exercise are just habits. Start slowly and avoid punishing for those inevitable slips. Forgive and go on. Plan little rewards along the way: go ahead and take a trip, or see a show, or buy those great shoes (preferably running shoes).

Remember: Any successful weight management plan must include the correct balance among all food groups that can be sustained for a lifetime. It has to include

EMOTIONS OF THIRTIES WOMEN

. . . .

- ❦ Worry about not having enough time to get everything done
- ❦ Excitement about who I am and what I have to say
- ❦ Satisfaction with finding my voice, looking good and sounding good
- ❦ Anxiety about my falling energy level
- ❦ Worry about others and how to keep everyone happy
- ❦ Wondering how long I have before I start to look older
- ❦ Desire for an active sex life and intimacy with my partner
- ❦ Ambivalence about my biological clock, children and my career
- ❦ My career is important but I feel torn between my family and my job

see sidebar next page

readily available foods, some favorite foods, and foods that fit both budget and lifestyle. Most important, it must include regular enjoyable exercise.

The American obsession with weight is fascinating. The average American woman is 5 feet 4 inches tall, weighs 140 pounds, and wears a size 14. The so-called "ideal" woman — portrayed by models, Miss America, Barbie dolls, and screen actresses — is 5 feet 7 inches, weighs 100 pounds, and wears a size 8.

One-third of all American women wear a size 16 or larger, and 75 percent of American women are dissatisfied with their appearance. Half of American women are on a diet at any one time. Between 90 percent and 99 percent of reducing diets fail to produce permanent weight loss. Two-thirds of dieters regain the weight within one year. Virtually all regain it within five years.

In fact, in the United States, just about every woman is concerned about weight on some level. All realize the pounds come on easier and come off harder. They may wish their metabolism would speed back up, or mourn the struggle to lose that five pounds that used to melt off in a week, or wonder if they'll ever lose baby weight. Many battle the discouragement and self-hatred of chronic obesity.

The weight-loss industry has successfully placed weight loss front and center in female consciousness. Models 20 years ago weighed eight percent less than the average woman. Today the gap has tripled and they weigh 23 percent less! Not surprisingly, shedding unwanted weight is on the minds of most Thirties Women, all the more so with attention on the "growing epidemic" of obesity. This focus on weight has so distorted women's views of themselves that in one study, three out of four women stated that they were overweight although only one out of four actually were.

Although avoiding obesity is a prudent strategy at any age, most women's weight concerns are based on body image rather than health concerns. Despite her athleticism, Angela's motivation for dropping those pounds is really to look better rather than to improve her health. This is especially troublesome if young mothers allow their obsession with weight to prevent them from gaining enough weight while they are pregnant. They may also restrict their children's calorie consumption such that they cannot grow properly.

BALANCING WORK, FAMILY, AND SELF

Throughout history, women have always worked, and families have always depended on their earnings. They continue to do so today. The aproned domestic divas of the 1950s were an anomaly, created by the need to remove women from the post-World War II economy and provide jobs for returning veterans. Although the need for women to work has changed little, women's expectations—both of themselves and their families—have changed a lot.

Although Angela's sister feels driven to make a difference as a physician, Angela — and millions of women like her — is a mother who works by financial necessity. Michelle, on the other hand, is a working mother driven by a personal and creative need to work. Michelle's commitment to marriage

EMOTIONS OF THIRTIES WOMEN

- ❀ Worry about my health and my changing body
- ❀ Worry that something will happen to the people I love
- ❀ Worry that I might die and leave my children alone
- ❀ Excitement about all the possibilities in my life
- ❀ Eager to get going in new directions
- ❀ Guilt that I want more time for myself
- ❀ Puzzled about where I am in all of this and who I am

HOW TO FIND A MENTOR

. . . .

- ❀ Join a professional or networking organization and watch for women in your field of interest who want to share their expertise.

- ❀ Call the library and ask for a list of clubs for women, including philanthropic organizations.

- ❀ Ask friends or family members if they know a woman who could be a resource.

- ❀ Start a mentoring program in your company and invite mentors and women seeking mentors. Bring everyone to the table and plan to be happy with the results.

and motherhood has not erased her commitment to her career. She perceives herself as a professional woman who loves her business, for which she has worked *very* hard and sacrificed much. It forms a vital portion of her self-image. In contrast, Lisa's primary focus is her family. She would never return to work if the family economy could survive without her income. Jennifer loves her work and has poured much of her life's energy into her career; so much so, in fact, that she worries about ever having a family.

Mentors—whether family members or not — help a lot with aging, personal development, and careers. Without a mentor, Thirties Women may view women currently in their seventies, eighties, and nineties as frighteningly old. Women who have had close relationships with such older women are less likely to be frightened by what is ahead of them.

Older role models are so important, and we found that women really want to know what their age mates think and how they are doing with the "aging thing." Our Thirties Women will make wonderful mentors because they have so much to share with younger women who are still trying to answer the question: "What do I want to be when I *really* grow up?" Women with good career successes can usually list a supportive and involved mentor, good role models, and a good support system as important factors helping them advance. It's interesting that this support comes from men at least as often as from other women.

By the same token, women who struggle in their careers often lacked this advantage. These women said it was difficult to find good mentors to help them with career choices and concerns. Whether they don't know where to look, don't know how to ask, or lack the personality traits to make such a relationship work, finding mentors and female role models seems to be a problem for some women.

All four of our Thirties Women could have used a mentor. It would have eased Jennifer's struggles with proving her youth and gender to her older male co-workers. Angela needs help re-structuring her career for sustainability and increased income into her later years. Michelle needs to learn how to handle her own financial affairs and run the money side of her business. Lisa needs to make a smooth and profitable workforce reentry after her youngest goes to school.

Another factor that limits the opportunity to find a mentor is that some women feel too much competition to help each other. This is unfortunate, because a woman truly has nothing to gain and everything to lose by stomping on the hands of another woman as she tries to climb the ladder. Some hyper-competitive women may have advanced through playing the men's game and have taken over the role of great oppressor. Others may just be too insecure or frightened to give advice, share worries, or reassure each other they are normal. People who manage all-female offices often complain about how bitchy and backbiting women can be. Such women usually feel powerless, so the bitchiness may stop if they feel empowered. All of these factors should make each of us more sensitive to young women who ask our advice.

The lucky ones have girlfriends with whom they can commiserate. Relationships are vitally impor-

HOW TO BECOME A MENTOR

* Reach out to offer assistance to a woman in your professional organization or company.

* Consider the time spent mentoring, whether in a formal or informal fashion, as an investment in other women.

* Tell friends and family about your goal to mentor women in your field, and help make connections between others.

* Go to your company's human resources department or employee assistance group to see if there are any programs in place. If not, offer to help create one.

HOW NOT TO FEEL INVISIBLE IN YOUR THIRTIES

....

- 🌺 Strut your stuff. Enter the room full of joy and anticipation, smile, and they will wonder what you have been up to.

- 🌺 Cultivate your sense of humor and personality. If you show genuine interest in others, no one will be able to forget you.

- 🌺 Be spontaneous. Trust your instincts and let your great ideas and dreams out to play.

- 🌺 Take time for your personal needs: get a new hairdo, learn a skill, study a new language, or take up a hobby. Have you always wanted to learn to shoot? Get a concealed weapons license, join a gun club that offers classes, and buy yourself a pearl-handled Derringer.

tant to women of every age, and whatever their specific needs, our Thirties Women were ready to be done with dating. They had purposefully moved on to finding (or keeping) their mate and growing their family. Those who want children are feeling a sense of urgency.

These young women take for granted that they should be able to do any job, pursue any dream. They stare in disbelief when they hear older women's tales of past gender discrimination.

FINDING HER TRUE SELF

In their twenties, women grow used to seeing images of themselves everywhere in advertising campaigns: young, lovely, unlined. Most of the people marketing products and writing scripts for television programming are young as well. Now, Thirties Women are moving rapidly into advertising limbo and it's much harder to find images of women who look like them on anything but ads for Botox or anti-aging treatments. Although they may be too busy to think about it consciously, on some level they feel left out and ignored.

Thirties Women may worry about their looks whether or not they have found a committed partner. Lisa has a loving and supportive husband yet she still employs fad diets and other extreme measures to keep her weight down, injections to combat wrinkles, and cosmetic surgery. Her husband really doesn't care — he loves her as she is — so, who is she doing this for? To look good in the eyes of other women? Or herself? For nearly one in five Thirties Women, their appearance is their biggest aging concern.

This concern with appearance can start very young. Girls of 16 have cosmetic surgery, already feeling at their young age the pressure to be physically and sexually appealing. I worry what these women will be doing when they reach their thirties, forties, and beyond, when the rate of cosmetic surgery increases markedly. In fact, 40 percent of all cosmetic procedures are done on women ages 30 to 50, years when women increasingly complain that they feel "invisible" and don't like it!

Thirties Women have no illusions about how much society values youth and beauty, and many are struggling to maintain their self-image. They see the double standard and say they wish that an aging woman would be viewed in the same way as an aging man, namely as sophisticated and wise. In reality, however, this is an unrealistic view of a man's experience. Men confront a host of anxieties and fears about aging that they mostly do not verbalize. But that's another story entirely.

Like Lisa, Angela, and Michelle, women commonly marry for the first time between ages 25 and 35. Like Angela, a lot of them also divorce before age 34. Thirties Women worry about their relationships, even if — or especially if — like Jennifer they have not yet found a partner. Family and settling down is a thirties concern and married women struggle with the challenges of changes in relationships they may have entered in their twenties.

Many women wait until their thirties to begin having children. Census statistics show that about 40 percent of first babies are born to women between the ages of 30 and 39. This group of women has seen mothers and other female role models having careers and families and doing a good job at both. They seize their right to have choices about kids, family, and work. Still, they agonize about whether they have made the right choice and whether they are doing a good job. There's just never enough time.

. . . .

Don't sweat the small stuff. The alternative to
aging gracefully is aging like a whining hag!

. . . .

Most of them have by now put aside their concerns about finding (or creating) the "perfect" mate. Still, Thirties Women think a lot about keeping their committed relationships. They express it in various ways: "Will we stay together? Is this the right partner or relationship for me? Can I keep this wonderful mate I found? Is this the one I can spend my life with? Do I still want to be with this

THINGS THIRTIES WOMEN WISH OTHERS UNDERSTOOD ABOUT THEM

. . . .

- ❀ How important my career is to me.
- ❀ It is hard for me to sacrifice my career and friends for my family's needs.
- ❀ I feel tired all the time.
- ❀ I feel confused about the changes in my body.
- ❀ It is hard for me to depend on a man.
- ❀ I worry about failing my family, my work, and my community.
- ❀ I don't want people to find out that I am not as caring as I should be.
- ❀ I am scared that I'll make poor decisions about my family's well-being.
- ❀ I worry that I will be found out as a fake who is plagued by constant doubts.
- ❀ I feel guilty that sometimes I want to run away and leave it all behind.

person for the rest of my life? Does he still love me even if I'm not as sexual as I once was? Am I still pleasing my mate?"

Dating is the major concern for the one-third of Thirties Women who are still (or again) single. When they wake in the night, Angela and Jennifer ask: "Will I find someone who will accept me as I age? Am I building a good family? Can I find a spouse to be my best friend, and grow old happily together?"

Thirties Women know that strong support systems are crucial to their futures and their well-being whether they have coupled or are single women or single parents. These women grew up in a time when group dates were the norm. Crowds of young people would meet at the mall for a movie rather than pairing off in couples like earlier generations, so many of them have tight circles of friends. Married or single, they know that strong ties to others enrich their emotional, psychological, and spiritual lives. With such support, women no longer feel the need to rush into second marriages when they perceive there are other ways to find companionship and trusting relationships.

Thirties Women are coming to terms with who they really are. They worry about what others will think and about whether they are doing things right. If they can hold hands with their sisters, they will discover more answers, compare notes, and help guide each other through this foreign territory.

"Seize the Day" is their watchword, although they express it in many different ways: "Make sure you live every day to its fullest. Try and do everything that you've been even the littlest bit curious about, and you'll have no regrets. Don't wait for tomorrow, until after the kids are gone, after that next big break at work, or after you retire to enjoy life. Live each moment like it is your last and enjoy your family."

Dr. Nancy's Kick-Butt Keys for Thirties Women

- Make peace with how far you have come in your career, and how much you earn.
- Let go of feeling judged by your peers.
- Nurture your newly emerging self-confidence and stronger spirituality.
- Take better care of yourself to retain your energy, vital glow, and healthy size.
- Choose relationships based on mutual interest and support.
- Pay attention to your body and screen for early signs of disease.
- Cherish and build strong support systems of extended family and friends.
- Find a mentor or be a mentor.
- Learn to manage finances; spend less and earn more so you can invest.
- Live every day to the fullest.

Thirties Women have high expectations for themselves and others. Their Super Mom fantasies are alive and well. They have gained confidence as they moved out of their twenties, and they have a treat in store when they pass into their forties.

Visit www.womenspeak.com to learn more about the thirties. Express yourself and share ways you have learned, grown, and found your best life.

CHAPTER 4

The 40s
Stop the Clock—I Wanna
Get Off!

We celebrated our last child going off to college by running
naked through the house!

SARA, 40

The Forties Woman is at the literal midpoint of her life. A woman who celebrates her forty-first birthday today can expect to live at least another 41 years to become 82. Many will live much longer. Actuarial projections aside, women in this decade may have a distinct impression of time accelerating — and bringing sweeping changes to every aspect of their lives.

The Forties Woman feels ambivalent. Should she try to stay young or should she just accept the passage of years? She struggles with myriad changes — in her body, her family roles, her intimate relationships, and her self-image. What helps a Forties Woman feel successful is to know her strengths and believe in her ability to directly affect her own life. At 40, women are starting to use the life lessons learned at younger ages — the importance of a good diet, an exercise regime, personal and professional goals, and an action plan. Keeping a positive attitude, accepting a realistic view of herself, and staying connected with other people will help the Forties Woman succeed.

One crucial thing that all Forties Women agreed on is the tremendous value of sharing their life experiences with other women. Finding a mentor and becoming a mentor are useful moves any woman can make. By talking with women who are older than ourselves, we learn that our views on aging are all relative and that our perspectives will change with the passing years. By talking with younger women, we can pass on the relief of knowing that others have had similar experiences and that we are not crazy.

WHAT FORTIES WOMEN WORRY ABOUT

Many Forties Women — more than 40 percent — are afraid of getting older. That's a lot of fear, although it's a lower percentage than in women in their twenties and thirties. The Forties Women profiled here represent a wide range of attitudes and experiences. Louise and Julia are afraid of getting older; Kathy and Marlene are not. Although these women have a great deal in common, they differ in important ways. The ones who fear aging worry much more about their appearance and are more likely to list "self" as their primary aging concern than the ones who are not fearful. Women who are not afraid tend to accept life's changes, to focus more on the benefits and joys of getting older, and to think about the impact their aging will have on their families and children.

Women say they fear growing older for a variety of reasons. Nearly a third of Forties Women say their biggest aging concern is their health. More than a fourth say their primary concern was money. Only 14 percent of Forties Women say their main concern as they get older is their appearance, and only a tenth of them say their main aging concern was family or being alone without a mate. Forties Women have gotten it together, and not even one says her major aging concern is her psychological or emotional wellbeing.

As they enter this time of reflection, Forties Women appreciate their own accomplishments and growing confidence. Yet they all express dismay that society seems to place so little value on their experience. This sense of being devalued frustrates and enrages women.

MARLENE: "I LIKE MYSELF BETTER NOW THAT I HAVE LESS SELF-DOUBT."

"Excellent therapy helped me overcome my anxiety about finding another husband," says Marlene, 40, who is divorced and has no children. Coming through the fire of divorce has made her stronger and more confident of her ability to take care of herself.

Marlene has plenty of dates and is comfortable taking a lover — or not. Since her divorce, she's as likely to direct her energies into her work, athletics, and art hobbies. "I have so many friends and activities in my life that bring me joy, it's really OK to live alone. I learned to love and honor myself after it dawned on me that I didn't have to wait for a man to make my dreams come true."

Unlike some of her friends who are battling "Forties Fatigue," Marlene feels more energetic and vital than ever. "I am so happy that I don't have to start from scratch," she says, giving thanks to her parents for their positive example. "I'm grateful their healthy habits rubbed off on me." Good problem-solving skills helped her modify her already solid diet and exercise program to fit her slower forties metabolism. Fad diets and quick fixes held no appeal, because she had seen them fail her friends time after time. "When I talk with other women who are successfully staying in shape, they say that having an action plan and goals for themselves makes the difference."

Since Marlene was never a big contender in the beauty competition, she thinks women waste the time and money they devote to trying to make them- selves beautiful. "You will always see yourself as less attractive than others see you, so you should forget about being perfect and just enjoy what you have. Beauty is, after all, subjective, and I believe I have done pretty well with what I have."

Philosophical about her appearance, Marlene does not buy the cosmetic industry's hype. While other women glance furtively at the magazines displayed at the grocery checkout and try to memorize which product promises which amazing benefit, Marlene laughs at their silliness.

·································

*Women can find balance in looking beneath the
surface and being happy the way they are.*

·································

Knowing what the future is likely to bring, she wants to squeeze all the enjoy- ment she can out of the present. "I realize that in 20 years, I'll probably be at least 10 pounds heavier, my breasts will be two inches lower, and I'll be losing my hair. So I think, "Wow, I'm beautiful now."

Marlene has worked hard to develop her positive attitude, and has paid a bundle for years of therapy she believes helped her a lot. "There's a high cost to embracing your own vulnerability," she laughs. "The pay-back has been a dramatic shift in the way I see myself. Ten years ago I was fearful and shy, always expecting to be judged.

"I never used to approach others unless they spoke first," she recalls. "Then I realized everyone's as scared as I am. Here's my revelation: Nobody is scrutinizing me as much as I feared."

As she struggled to find her voice and courage, she uses quotes and affirmations: "Comfort is not a requirement," and "Life shrinks or expands in proportion to one's courage."

Equally important to her growth has been forging more connections with women friends and relatives as mentors and in groups. This has helped her counter one of the more painful realities of aging, Marlene says: the sense that women lose societal support. "I find it sad that our society seems to be moving toward increasing superficiality, and that older people are not valued and revered for their wisdom and for what they've survived."

Although she believes a social network is important to successful aging, Marlene says a woman must ultimately take personal responsibility for her experience. "Women need to stand up and stop allowing Madison Avenue to dictate how they feel about aging. We need to be proud of our maturity and what we have contributed to society. Until we stop acting like aging is a curse, it will remain a curse."

When others complain about losing the attention they enjoyed in their youth, she says earnestly, "I used to feel invisible when I held back my thoughts, feelings, ideas, and opinions, or was with people who judged me harshly. Now I feel good about myself when I respond to others and they respond to me. I feel heard."

Marlene remembers that she always enjoyed her parents' friends, and she has reached out to include older women at her parties. Some of her guests have expressed surprise by the inclusion of elders, but she believes women cheat themselves if they don't open up their social circles. "I hope that at 49 I am young and at 100 will still be young at heart," Marlene says. Despite her affirming attitude toward aging, Marlene's comments show she, too, thinks of being young as the positive and being old as the negative.

Still, Marlene says, "I hope to enjoy being me, just as I am. I've been getting there for the past few years as I've worked through my anxieties, and the process has clarified for me what's really important: I'm important." For a woman who has spent most of her life catering to the needs of others, the idea of her own importance is a revelation. By conquering her fears and learning to see beyond herself with a clear eye, she has learned to connect with others and accept and believe their kind words.

Although she strives to be compassionate, Marlene has little patience with women who wallow in self-pity about getting older. "My attitude is, 'I feel your pain — now move on!'" To maintain her youthful spirit, she does at least one new thing each year, preferably something she's been afraid to do before. "It doesn't have to be anything dramatic or dangerous; it could be something simple, like tasting rutabagas." Her key is to keep an open mind, expand her comfort zone, and see things from a fresh perspective.

In some ways, Marlene admits, she actually likes growing older. "I like myself better now that I have less self-doubt. I have finally committed to living free of negative people and my own negative self-talk. Now I worry less about growing old than about making the most of each day and appreciating it."

. . . .

SO MANY WOMEN HAVE A hard time accepting their own power and talents and don't believe they can affect their worlds. But Marlene did just that, with a vengeance! Her life-changing event — a divorce — presented an opportunity to take charge. Marlene became her own champion through her difficult divorce.

Many women feel isolated and guilt-ridden because they take sole responsibility for the failure of a marriage. They find it hard to re-enter a social world so they withdraw. Marlene said, "No way." Knowing her looks would not be her drawing card, she realistically assessed her strengths: her personality, her ability to make friends, and her ability to develop plans. These enabled her to find the comfort and support that helped her stay connected with her world. She also used a good mental health professional, an excellent investment for any person whose life suddenly takes a left turn even though their right turn signal is on.

Everyone has fears of aging and dying, and it's natural to think of being young as more attractive and appealing than being old. Our society exerts strong pressure in support of this belief. However, we don't have to allow ourselves to be debilitated by that fear. One useful step is to notice the way we think about ourselves and about our lives as the years pass, and then re-frame it. Take time to cruise your favorite bookstore's Self-help and Women's Issues sections. Notice how many volumes focus on stopping the clock to stay young. Now there's a losing game! Surely we will benefit more by finding ways to become mature, attractive, and exciting women at forty, fifty, or sixty and beyond.

Marlene discovered to her pleasure that she could reap the rewards from her own actions and feel pride in her own accomplishments. She found her power through "ownership" of her ability to affect her world directly, and now is confident of her abilities. Psychologists say women like Marlene have a great "locus of control." They feel in charge of their fate instead of buying lottery tickets or hoping that a rabbit's foot pays off. They are their own agents of change and say, "Come on world, let's get it on." They sleep well at night and wake with the knowledge that they are in charge of their own lives.

As Marlene's example illustrates, women can take charge of their lives. They can accept both the responsibility and the fruits of their labors and come out feeling powerful. Marlene is taking personal responsibility for her feelings and experiences, getting professional assistance to help her grow and succeed.

A woman who makes her own luck and plans her future can expect to be successful. The power of positive thinking, good self-image, and staying connected and realistic about oneself will help ensure success. These confident women know they do not need someone to complete them; they are already a good package. In her basket of resources a woman like Marlene has included the many friends and activities that get her out in the world and connected. She seeks support and guidance and gains energy from these resources. She has found her power and learned ways to overcome her shyness. Marlene realized that her isolation and withdrawal kept her frightened and feeling out of control, so she seized control and put herself on the top of her Very Important People list. Marlene demonstrates that loving yourself leads to a healthier worldview and paves the way for a healthy adjustment even after a devastating loss such as a divorce or death.

Marlene also has learned that having a good diet, an exercise regime, an action plan, and personal and professional goals makes her feel like a winner. Marlene views her life in terms of opportunities and possibilities, and she now expects to win. And why not? Marlene has learned these important life lessons quite young.

I can say without reservation that Marlene is on the right road. She has a great road map for her journey and she has all her bags packed with the right stuff. She knows that although her road may have a few bumps and potholes, she has the keys to her car and her own AAA membership if she has a problem. Marlene is a survivor and will make a great mentor for other women of all ages.

JULIA: "NON-BREEDING WOMEN ARE REGARDED AS SUPERFLUOUS."

Julia, 46, is reasonably satisfied with her work as an accountant. Unlike Marlene, she is afraid of getting older. She has never married nor had children. This leaves her feeling excluded in her Midwestern community, where she says "non-breeding women are regarded as superfluous." She's had good advancement on the job, and, conscious of the need to support herself, she has maintained a tight budget and put money away for her retirement. "Too many women spend their lives taking care of others and make no provisions for themselves."

Julia is among a growing number of women who focus on their careers. They aren't driven by the ticking of their biological clocks and prefer to develop their professional and financial strengths rather than build a family.

Despite her career success and her physical attractiveness, Julia is plagued by insecurity and jealousy. "I think about getting older most often when I see my boyfriend talking to another woman," Julia says. "We've been together for almost two years and don't see anyone else. He says he loves me and that he appreciates my quiet personality and life perspective, and that it's refreshing to spend time with someone who is interesting and thoughtful. I just wish I did not wonder if he still thinks that when he is talking to another woman, especially one who is younger."

Julia's mother never discussed her aging process, although she fought it every inch of the way, and drank heavily to hide from the reality. Menopause might as well have been a forbidden topic; it was simply never discussed. Consequently, when Julia hit perimenopause early, she had no idea what was happening to her or how to cope. "It was not a happy, rose-filled adventure," Julia recalls. "It was a rocky horror show in hell."

The one time Julia gathered her courage and tried to learn about what was happening to her, she had little success. "I asked my doctor for information to help me through the menopause process," she says. "All he offered me was a flier from a hormone manufacturer." When she asked her mother for advice about dealing with menopause, her mother replied only, "Be glad when it's over."

Although she had initially feared menopause, now that she is nearly there, her fears are dissipating. With greater or lesser grace, she has started to adjust her expectations. Rather than torturing herself to achieve her ideal weight, she now seeks to keep her weight under control. Rather than constantly striving to look great, she has developed a professional look that fits her career goals.

....

My mother has a permanent spot in her plastic surgeon's parking lot and I have toyed with the idea of a facelift.

....

That's progress, and helps reassure her she won't end up like her mother, who she says runs from aging like a maniac. "My mother has a permanent spot in her plastic surgeon's parking lot and I have even toyed with the idea of a facelift. I guess on some level, I am still my mother's child. I worry that when I hit her age, I may be just as unhappy and angry as she is."

Lately, Julia has grieved that her relationship with her mother has not grown warmer and deeper. Her mother has always taken a stoic approach to life, never talking about her feelings about aging and even denying her many cosmetic surgeries. To her mom, personal matters are messy, embarrassing, and best kept to oneself.

This has left Julia feeling bereft because she believes a loving family would show their feelings. She envies women who have a good support group and family members that love them for who they are without asking them to change. One indication of her deep sense of lack is that she does not expect to ever have that for herself.

Because Julia is afraid of aging, she's having an especially hard time accepting it, and she feels essentially alone. "I wish I had a circle of women friends with common interests," says Julia, who is too shy to have developed many friendships. If people in general, and particularly women, had discussed such matters from the time of her youth, she believes menopause might have been less of a shock. If women would talk about the natural changes that come as they age, they could help each other a lot and it would make the hormonal changes less fearsome.

Julia says bitterly that society sees menopausal women as "withered empty vessels waiting to die." This makes her angry, and she wishes aging women could behave — and be treated — like wise elders who deserve respect. Instead, she sees them as isolated and lonely. Sometimes Julia feels depressed. Her mother has depression, and she assumes this is her lot as well.

Although Julia has considered plastic surgery, she knows in her heart it won't remove the root of her fear, which stays hidden except at night. "When I go to bed, I think about my mortality, and the fear paralyzes me. I want to be able to choose when I die. I do not want to be a vegetable in a nursing home with no family to take care of me." Julia's experiences with the health professions have left her without a shred of trust in any of them. Women who feel they have little support and are used to giving rather than receiving tend to worry a lot about self-care and being a burden to others. This is especially common in women like Julia who have bypassed marriage and children.

"I've always been shy, and these days when I'm in a group, I often feel ignored and unheard," says Julia. Although this has been increasing in her forties, she says it doesn't really bother her all that much. As she gets older, she finds strength in being quiet and listening. Watching others posture to grab attention amuses her. More important to her now is her sense of personal integrity; she prides herself on honoring her commitments.

· ·

ALTHOUGH JULIA'S "VOICE" IS A quiet one, accepting that fact does not make her feel invisible. As women like Julia move through their forties they gain confidence and trust in themselves. With grace and style, they find their "groove" and realize that they like the women they have become. For Julia, part of learning who she is has been the development of a strong sense of purpose and spirituality. When women find themselves they often also find a higher power to comfort and guide them to inner peace.

One of Julia's greatest challenges is that she has not yet found a role model to show her what "successful aging" looks like. Her mother focused her time and money on trying to beat the clock. Julia got the message that getting older was frightening. She is insecure and constantly compares herself to other women and feels anxious about her ability to hold her man. Once her youthful bloom fades she expects to be alone and dismissed.

Most women have issues of some type about their appearance and many struggle with their self-image. Aging brings with it a loss of the youthful self, and many women experience a prolonged period of grieving that loss. It also brings a need to re-define who we are. She feels no support from her mother and — having chosen not to have children — she is concerned about ending up alone. Her greatest fear is that if she becomes ill and dependent she will have to rely on strangers to care for her.

Talking to other women is great medicine. Julia is yearning for a women mentor to help in her life and job. Such support from other women is key to many women's well-being and success. Julia's best chance to overcome her fears is to find a female mentor with whom she can talk about her concerns. So far, she has primarily noticed the women in her life who — like her mother — make every effort to stop time and to forestall aging. She's thinking about resorting to such remedies to keep herself young and beautiful. Because this nebulous goal is impossible to achieve, her self-worth may suffer further. In addition, she may experience bouts of depression, anxiety, and other health problems if she does not find constructive outlets for her fears. If she does not intervene, her fears of aging and envy of others' happiness could come to dominate her life as she continues to grow older.

Everyone gets the blues now and then, but ongoing depression is neither normal nor inevitable. Women can find the medical and psychological help they need to feel good about themselves and enjoy life. The hormone fluctuations of perimenopause take emotions on a roller coaster ride much like those of adolescence. Anxiety and the blues can develop and a woman's fears of losing beauty and energy can escalate into fears of losing her mind. Some women begin to experience full-blown anxiety attacks for the first time. Many women feel this way. It's so important that they express these feelings now.

It's critically important that women find healthcare providers and support systems to guide them through this painful and difficult transition. Knowledge is power, so any woman who is struggling with this needs to talk to her doctor and close friends whom she respects and knows will listen.

At this point, Julia's awareness and discomfort are actually a gift, a strength she can build on. If she pays attention, she can begin to make changes now and take a detour around those feelings of being unwanted and unloved. She is comfortable doing her own financial planning and has built her earning power and savings for self-sufficiency, so she can extend those skills to set up a plan for her own old age.

In addition, one good way to counter her fear of having to rely on strangers is to develop friendships. In fact, many women have created their own intentional families in which they give and receive loving support. By working to develop a support system she could pay more attention to making her remaining days full of life instead of focusing on her final end. This will help her relationships, too, because even if they end — and many will — she'll have a support system and other activities to sustain her.

However, becoming ill and helpless is Julia's primary concern. Fortunately she has the resources to buy long-term care insurance, and she needs to investigate the many extended care products that the insurance industry is rapidly developing. It also might relieve her fears to research long-term care facilities in her area — and even to those at some distance. An increasing number of places offer independent and assisted living with the option of nursing care in the context of thriving communities of seniors.

Finally, and most important, Julia is matching her faith in herself with a growing belief in a higher power that she can draw upon for guidance. Finding a comfortable church community could help her feel less alone. Women say that faith in a higher power helps them adjust to life's challenges and gives them strength in difficult times.

Instead of lying in bed at night with her Stinken Thinken, obsessing about her eventual death, Julia could take control. Noticing that she is doing this is the first step, which she has already taken. Next, she should journal these thoughts so she can look at them objectively and see what part of this she can do something about. None of us can foretell our future and most of our worries never come to pass. If she continues to struggle with these thoughts, she could learn to meditate or pray and shift her focus to gratitude.

She has much to be grateful for and much to share with others. She possesses a strong desire to live in a fair and balanced world and could easily reach out to become a mentor herself. She has no trouble taking responsibility for herself and prides herself on being accountable for her actions. She is on a healthy path of awareness and has an opportunity to face the coming years with confidence and security.

I can't emphasize enough how important it is that Julia is aware of her feelings and wants to change them. Many women have not yet come to any level of awareness and therefore may find themselves depressed, anxious, and without a clue as to why they feel this way. Julia is ahead of the game because she has a strong sense of what does not feel right to her at this time in her life.

LOUISE: "I'VE LOST MY SENSE OF ENDLESS POSSIBILITIES."

At age 48, Louise feels powerful and more confident than ever that she can take care of her own needs. She has worked hard to advance her career and now heads a personnel department where she feels respected, if not necessarily well paid. Her husband, also a middle manager, appreciates her financial contribution to the family. All three kids are doing all right in school, seem reasonably well adjusted, and are becoming more independent every day. She thanks God that so far her parents' health is holding up.

Despite her overall self-confidence, lately she has been on an emotional roller coaster. A hysterectomy pushed her into menopause overnight and she crashed head-on into perimenopausal symptoms. She wants to understand how to deal with them, but no one she knows talks about it. "Although I know age is just a number, some days I feel like 70 or 80," she says. "One evening I started to make a joke about my hot flashes and just bit my tongue — I felt ashamed. Do others feel this way? Why doesn't anyone talk about it?"

. . . .

I started dyeing my hair and searching
for ways to feel sexy again.

. . . .

One of Louise's worst moments was when her husband said she was starting to look like her mother. She was crushed! "I started dyeing my hair and searching for ways to feel sexy again." Each time she looked in the mirror she saw more and more of her mother — *not* a comfortable experience.

The fact that Louise considers her mother (her closest role model) to be very old and sitting on life's sidelines does nothing to ease her concerns. "My mother complains about getting old, about her physical limitations, and that she's slipping mentally," Louise says. "She feels life passing her by and hates it, especially because she has done everything she could to stay young."

With her surgical menopause, Louise's sexual desire crashed along with her self-image, but she enjoys sex when her husband — whom she truly loves —

initiates it. Although she can barely admit it even to herself, she is also a bit anxious about keeping his interest. After 20-plus years of marriage, she trusts him — of course — yet the thoughts, "Does he still think I'm sexy?" and even occasionally "Is he running around on me?" flash through her consciousness.

Louise's experience is a common one for Forties Women experiencing what can be drastic hormonal, physical, and emotional changes. Many mature and successful women like Louise have built their careers, reared their children, nurtured good relationships, and feel confident and capable. Yet they feel stunned to find that a little thing like declining estrogen production can create such confusion and frustration. It has brought many a strong woman temporarily to her knees! The emotional ups and downs make it even harder to cope with the skin changes, wrinkles, fading vision, and other signs of growing older, not to mention the appalling weight gain!

Always considered pretty, Louise used to receive lots of attention for her looks. Now, she's grieving the loss of her ability to turn heads. Like most women her age, she cringes at the inescapable wrinkles, age spots, and gray hair. She mourns the loss of the power over others conferred by beauty and youth, but reminds herself that she is gaining wisdom and power over herself. She admits wistfully, "I wish I could look like I'm 40 when I am 60, and have known what I'll know at 60 when I was 40.

"I don't think our society likes us all that much — the attitude is so patronizing," Louise says. "I would like society to stop glamorizing young women all the time. I don't want to be 25 again. I want to be appreciated for being 48.

"The media should accentuate the inner beauty of the people they place in the limelight," Louise grumbles. "A woman is only as beautiful as she acts." She would like to see models of all ages and sizes, and have the attention focus on character and attitude.

Louise fears her aging will be a descent into illness and loss, and the changes in her body frighten her. When she thinks about getting older, which she does often, she worries about disease, and loss of functioning, and losing her emotional connections. "I'm afraid of being unloved or being unlovable, and not being able to give love to other people or to help other people," she says. Even so, she doesn't often worry about the effects of her aging on the people she loves, nor does she fret much about losing loved ones.

Her aging fear is "I don't want to be left behind," and she has worked to become more assertive and find her voice. That makes her feel strong and capable, but other times Louise catches herself trying to look and act younger. "I hate that!" she says. "It doesn't fool anybody, and I lose all the wonderful feelings and experiences of being the age I am."

She remembers as a teenager watching her mother's friends. "One of them wore miniskirts and tall leather boots, like my friends and I wore. One day I saw her bend over to pick up her coat and I promised myself that when I got old I would not make that mistake. I haven't worn a miniskirt since my teens, but I *do* like the tall boots."

Louise saw for herself that trying to beat the clock can in fact backfire. Her memory banks store these negative images and her inner voice tells her: "Act your age!" But what exactly does that mean? A Katherine Hepburn look or a Joan Rivers look? Louise has focused her energies on cultivating her own unique look and finding ways to like herself and her accomplishments.

Even more than changes in her appearance, Louise's loss of energy has changed her outlook on life. She says wistfully, "I've lost my sense of endless possibilities, the sense that I can always do something different, take on a major self-directed change. I just don't have the energy." Feeling this decline makes her even more anxious about being able to work and care for herself and her family as she grows older.

In my clinical practice I saw many women like Louise who wondered why they were exhausted all the time. Seeing themselves as "Dr Mom," they had given at the office, given to the community, volunteered at their church, and then fixed a gourmet dinner for a romantic night at home with their significant other. They would drive themselves relentlessly, yet were surprised to hear that they had good reason to be exhausted. I encouraged them to re-evaluate and re-write their job descriptions.

At least partly because of the pressure she places on herself, Louise has already developed multiple health issues. She takes medicines for insomnia, depression, and migraines. She knows women who have fibromyalgia and chronic pain and worries she might develop these as well. "Can one afford to be ill anymore?" she asks. "And even if you can afford care, who is going to look after you without abusing you? I worry about becoming a nonentity, physically unable to take care of myself."

Louise occasionally daydreams about retiring with leisure to spoil her grand-children and enjoy her life. She wonders how much it would cost to live in a retire-ment community, but those ideas have little reality for her. She and her husband spend most of what they earn each year on their family, and haven't been able to put much away for their future.

Their investment in parenting their rebellious teens is finally paying off, and their children are emerging as young adults who are fun to be with. "We are really beginning to enjoy each other's company," Louise says. "We took a trip to the beach and just hung out. I am going to like being friends with my grown kids."

. . . .

FORTIES WOMEN LIKE LOUISE OBSERVE their physical changes, aging parents, and emptying nests and are taking stock. Some work to re-kindle love affairs with their husbands and some are considering other alternatives. Many of them for the first time realize they can design a path for themselves. They can look at the "me" instead of the "we." During this middle-aged preparation a woman can consider how she wants her next decades to unfold. Increasingly, Forties Women are letting go of the self-defeating goal of filling everyone's needs but their own.

Louise exemplifies the many changes of the forties and the emergence of new issues to consider. She reacted to her husband's comments that she looked like her mother by fearing he would no longer find her desirable. Although many women experience a temporary drop in sexual desire, for many others their sexual satisfaction becomes more important when they no longer worry about pregnancy. This is many women's first opportunity to consider sex as an outlet and an expression of intimacy with their partner. Sex for sex's sake offers new rewards for a mature, confident empty-nester interested at last in her own needs. Yet this is another double bind for Forties Women, because at the same time they worry that their bodies are becoming less sexy.

Forties Women who have good female role models for successful aging are better prepared and more comfortable with their own aging than those who do not. Louise, like the many women who did not have a successful model in a friend or family member, feels ill prepared.

Louise has watched her mother's futile struggle with aging and hopes to avoid a similar experience. She has seen older women refuse to change their clothing and behavior and has added the term "age-appropriate" to her vocabulary. She feels embarrassed when her mother acts like an aging teen, yet Louise often feels little older than a teenager herself. This is a confusing time for Forties Women because the way they feel inside may get increasingly out of step with the way their bodies look.

Women who believe on some level that their appearance is the source of their identity, will fear losing their looks *and* their man. Louise's feeling of vulnerability causes her mind and her body to send out distress signals in the form of loss of energy and depression. These in turn bring additional lethargy and lack of motivation to seek assistance.

Louise needs to find a good mentor, friend, or counselor, someone she can talk with. Too many women sit silently with their fears of aging, all the while thinking they are the only one struggling. Some of them do not want to burden others with their concerns; other falsely assume that everyone else is doing fine.

Women in their forties are smart to take a serious look ahead to re-inventing themselves and to their eventual retirement if they have not already done so. Although Louise and her husband have not put much away for their futures, it is in no way too late for them to save and invest for retirement, travel, and leisure time with family and each other. By doing this, Louise also will teach her children the importance of planning ahead to ensure their needs will be met.

Her opportunity to re-invent herself is probably Louise's major resource and she can draw upon this to assist with aging issues in her forties and beyond. Although she may have lost her youthful sense of endless possibilities, she should open her eyes to the impressive range of options still available to a strong, skilled, and experienced woman of her caliber. A new look, a new job, new friends, and new interests are all within her grasp.

Louise's greatest challenge will be to better understand her fears and concerns about aging and losing her looks, which she equates with a personal failure and dismissal by her peers. Finding a role model, a mentor, and women with whom she can discuss her important questions will help her find the courage she needs.

KATHY: "WE NEED TO HANG TOGETHER AS WE AGE INTO RED-HOT MAMAS!"

Kathy, 49, left the workforce when she began having children in her twenties and has never returned. She looks back on her life so far with considerable satisfaction. She has dedicated her life to meeting her family's needs, and even when her children were small, she volunteered in her community.

She also devotes a lot of time to her friends and participates in several women's clubs. Here she has found friends who match her humor and spirituality and whom she admires. "For me it's important to have an integrated positive image as someone who is a good citizen, good mother, good marriage partner, and someone who can accept and appreciate what is around her," Kathy says.

It's from this group of varied girlfriends that she has learned how to deal with the stresses of getting older. "We all need to hang together as we age into Red Hot Mamas!" she says. Even though these friends support each other and joke about menopause, they rarely talk about the deepest levels of their fears and doubts. What she has learned about her own emotional, psychological, and physical changes, she has gathered from female voices in books, from lots of tough introspection, and from watching men who don't seem embarrassed by getting older.

One of the major benefits of her peer group has been realizing that — regardless of their personal styles and concerns — all her friends have wildly mixed emotions about getting older. Although her husband sometimes sulks a bit at the time she spends with her women friends, she refuses to be swayed. "I try to demonstrate my devotion to him and to our kids in other ways," she says.

She has talked with her friends about it, and they agree it's normal to feel a bit depressed now that her children are starting to leave home. "I feel stuck between two identities. Exactly who am I now? I like the freedom of having the children grown, but I miss nurturing them and feeling needed. What is my role now?" She feels emotional watching her children grow as she gets older herself.

Kathy hated having missed the Sixties and always considered herself something of an Earth Mother type. The prospect of getting older inspires Kathy to use the knowledge she has gained to build a happy life. Her plan is to grow continually, both spiritually and intellectually, and ultimately to take all her experiences and insights and do something worthy that will help others.

"I might have only thirty summers left to enjoy," she says. She is amazed and delighted to have few troubling perimenopause symptoms. "I wake up each day and count my blessings. I still have much wonder about this world and all the people populating it. I practice kindness, compassion, and inner peace. I like my searching mind and ability to learn.

"When I lay my hand next to my 20-year-old daughter's," says Kathy, "It reminds me of when I laid mine next to my mother's hands." Many positive feelings accompany these memories. "I have always respected older women," she says, "and I look forward to gaining wisdom, patience, and insight myself." Her aging concerns most often center on losing loved ones and not wanting to be a burden on her children. Beyond wondering, "Will I be in good health for my kids?" she rarely worries about illness.

Kathy has worked to cultivate her personality as much or more than her looks, and she's never been particularly vain. It's just as well, because she teaches a class at a community college and finds that being around young people presents several challenges. "It's harder to get attention and I am not noticed as much in groups as I used to be. The young, pretty women draw attention like a magnet, and not just from the young men." On the plus side, she's glad to be free of the pressure and insecurities of her twenties and thirties. She appreciates her new freedom and acknowledges a sense of passing the torch to younger women. She's most annoyed, however, by the disregard of some of these young people. "They'll assume I'm not interesting or that I won't understand an Internet procedure, or don't know a contemporary song. Because I enjoy older adults, for a long time I was the youngest in any group, but that's not true now and it never will be again."

....

Life is what we make it, so we must create our own quality of life as we want it to be. We can embrace every wrinkle and gray hair, and let our inner beauty shine through!

....

Kathy knows for sure that current standards of beauty are off base. "There is true beauty in a lined face. Those lines have been earned. It's a shame that they are not recognized as beautiful — even sadder that they must be a source of shame."

Despite that brave talk, she likes her own relatively unlined face (one benefit of the extra 20 pounds that arrived with her menopausal metabolism), and notes with a smile that she can always find someone who looks worse. Kathy's wishes for her future include continued good health and losing some weight, yet she focuses less on her appearance and more on feelings than Louise does. "I must accept the body God has given me; learn to love myself at each stage of life before I can love others. Aging is a natural process in life that I can either fight or accept with grace."

Women like Kathy have an easier time with aging because they accept themselves and refuse to define themselves by an age number. They have confidence in their ability to shape their own lives and maintain a young and vibrant attitude. Ultimately, women like Kathy believe that a woman ages well when she loves herself and doesn't depend on others for validation.

Self-sufficiency aside, one of her biggest challenges has been keeping her marriage interesting. "I want to keep the girl in the relationship yet still accept the old man he is becoming," she says. It was hard when she wasn't at all interested in sex for weeks at a time. "I love him, and don't want him to lose interest in me. I'd love to rekindle the love my husband had when we first married. Fortunately we've both been trying and I'm happy to report we're finding new intimacy and excitement."

Kathy's primary focus has been on raising her kids to be responsible, caring young people who respect their peers, elders, family, co-workers, the environment, and their country's leaders, Kathy says. "Yet sometimes I wonder 'Is this really all there is?' But then I think of those little kids turning into wonderful young adults!" She likes the feeling of becoming a real friend to her children and working with her husband to plan their future. In the present moment, however, they are consumed with their kids, making ends meet, and the increasing needs of aging parents and grandparents. "Seeing them become infirm is shaking me up," Kathy says. "Now I worry much more about my health than before and wonder if that will happen to me."

Watching her oldest child become an adult has made Kathy think of starting a life of her own again. When women in their forties shift the focus back on their own needs, they do so with a new maturity and calm. "I realized that I need to feel secure in myself first and in my relationships second," Kathy says. "That

PERIMENOPAUSE SYMPTOMS CAN INCLUDE:

. . . .

- ❀ Irregular periods
- ❀ Night sweats or insomnia
- ❀ Fatigue
- ❀ Loss of libido
- ❀ Emotional swings
- ❀ Irritability and sadness
- ❀ Weight gain
- ❀ Anxiety
- ❀ Vaginal dryness
- ❀ Mental fuzziness
- ❀ Lack of interest in favorite activities
- ❀ Feelings of hopelessness
- ❀ Fatigue and loss of energy
- ❀ Lack of motivation
- ❀ Feeling guilty or worthless for no reason
- ❀ Focusing on death or suicide
- ❀ Difficulty falling asleep or staying asleep

see sidebar next page

requires staying in touch with my own personal and emotional needs and filling them." She believes that age is primarily in the mind, so she has decided to keep learning and taking chances. Rather than becoming crystallized at one phase of her life, she lays claim to her inner self and pursues the things that interest her most.

When Kathy's youngest sister joined the Navy, her mother enrolled in college to finish her degree. "It was truly a wise decision," Kathy says. "My mom found she could still think, could still learn, and that she had lots of lifetime experiences to share with her classmates who were, in many instances, younger than her own kids. It was a great experience for her."

. . . .

FORTIES WOMEN LIKE KATHY ARE looking in the mirror and asking, "What do I really want to be when I grow up?" Kathy seems prepared and eager for change and sees it as her time. With her good health, family encouragement, and support from many friends, she is well on her way to finding real purpose and passion in the next phase of her life.

Women with attitudes and experiences like Kathy's cope very well with the physical and emotional changes of their forties. One of the best resources for successful aging is a determination to find one's passion and purpose. Kathy is on a positive path to do just that. She expects to be successful and regards her life experiences as a valuable commodity.

And why not? Kathy has much to look forward to. She is not hung up on her looks, has no regrets, and sees her life as being full of possibilities. She does not fear being alone nor does she expect obscurity or dismissal. On the contrary, she intends to grow and take on new challenges. These include reviving her sexuality and pumping romance and intimacy back into her relationship.

Women like Kathy also see their importance as mentors and teachers of the next generation. Her own children will learn from her the importance of making a difference. Kathy has faith in herself and her ability to age successfully. She sees her time on this earth as a gift. This leaves her little time to worry about looking or feeling old. Kathy has learned to love herself and regards aging as a natural process, not a disease.

As the stories of Marlene, Julia, Louise, and Kathy illustrate, each Forties Woman must weave her own life's tapestry out of the threads she inherits as well as those she spins for herself. Their quite different attitudes and life experiences, all of which fall well within the range of normal, influence the way they perceive this decade of tremendous change.

WHAT DO FORTIES WOMEN WANT?

One hundred years ago, the average woman didn't get a chance to worry about getting older. She died in her forties. Now a Forties Woman has another half of her life ahead of her. We are also being told that "Forty is the new thirty," so why wouldn't we think that our forties will be just another decade of youthful living before we begin the aging process?

So, what do Forties Women want? Their needs are different than when they were twenty or thirty,

PERIMENOPAUSE SYMPTOMS CAN INCLUDE:

. . . .

- ❀ Significant weight change
- ❀ Up to half of all women say they experience no negative symptoms at all during perimenopause

and they seek coping strategies. Perhaps more than anything else, women want to know if their physical changes, their emotions, their hopes, and their fears are normal. They are asking, "Am I doing this right or wrong? Can I do it better? What comes next?"

HEALTHY AND OH, SO HOT!

One thing that nearly all Forties Women want is help dealing with perimenopause and menopause. Many women say, "My mother never discussed menopause or getting older with me," and they are stunned to learn that perimenopausal signs can begin as early as their late twenties.

Overall, nearly every woman will begin to have irregular periods before she leaves her forties and many of them will have already reached menopause. Officially, menopause occurs in a woman's thirteenth month without a menstrual cycle. Although many women have times when they feel awful, many others breeze through perimenopause with few symptoms.

This passage can easily take 10 years, and many women are uninformed and frightened about this normal transition. What makes this worse is that menopause is not often discussed between mothers and daughters, or even girlfriends. Many women are not comfortable revealing their age, especially if they feel it threatens their job standing. In fact, as Julia discovered when her family doctor offered her a hormone pamphlet, it's often a dead-end topic even with a woman's healthcare provider. This leaves most women in the dark about what to do and where to turn for help. This silence can leave women who are frightened about aging — and may be worrying about their health for the first time — feeling even more confused and alone.

These women must learn to advocate for their own needs. They could seek out a different doctor who will listen and who will help with women's health issues such as perimenopause and menopause. It is possible to find a doctor who feels a special bond with women who are leaving their childbearing years. Some of these women waited to start a family and are shocked to discover they may not have enough eggs left to conceive a child. The window to conceive and bear a child closes earlier than they thought. Statisticians tell us that out of every 83 women who have a first baby, only four of them are between the ages of 40 and 44. There are additional risks involved with these late pregnancies as well.

Many women feel like they pass into medical oblivion once they stop ovulating. They may find themselves ignored, misunderstood, and invisible to healthcare professionals who are busy attending to women planning their next child. Even though many women are relieved and find their sex lives blossom once the fear of pregnancy is gone, they may have learned to feel used up or passed over once they leave their childbearing years. This happens because our society puts such a premium on being and staying young.

The roots of that belief extend far back in history. In ancient times, menopausal women were excluded from the privileges and leisure of the red tent, which was reserved for fertile females. Many women today feel embarrassed or ashamed without understanding why.

Although many women are not comfortable discussing it, most also have questions about their changing sexuality. Feeling used up or passed over definitely does not help a woman feel sexy. As a couple transitions into the empty nest phase, women need to unlearn these feelings if the relationship is to grow into greater intimacy and joy. Women who fear change in their relationships will miss out. In fact, many women in their forties do experience unimagined sexual freedom and may find excitement and lust in new or renewed relationships. "I had no idea how much fun I could have since my daughter left for college," says Jeanne, 44. "We act like lovesick puppies when we are alone and I am more satisfied than ever."

By the time perimenopause begins most women experience some changes in their desire and respon-

EMOTIONS OF FORTIES WOMEN

- ❋ Elation at fewer child responsibilities
- ❋ Anxiety about re-entering the workplace
- ❋ Grief at losing their nurturing role
- ❋ Fear of aging and illness
- ❋ Confusion about life goals
- ❋ Anticipation of new opportunity
- ❋ Disgust with body changes
- ❋ Exhaustion from sleep disturbance
- ❋ Joy in family closeness
- ❋ Envy of others who have it easier
- ❋ Happiness at being alive
- ❋ Anger at spouse or partner
- ❋ Mourning for loss of younger self
- ❋ Lust for new relationship
- ❋ Sorrow at lack of intimacy

COMMON SYMPTOMS OF DEPRESSION

. . . .

- ❀ Constant sadness
- ❀ Lack of motivation
- ❀ Irritability
- ❀ Trouble concentrating
- ❀ Hopelessness
- ❀ Feeling fatigued
- ❀ Loss of energy
- ❀ Feeling guilty or worthless
- ❀ Focusing on death or suicide
- ❀ Trouble sleeping
- ❀ Significant weight change
- ❀ Isolation from family and friends
- ❀ Lack of interest in favorite activities

siveness. Often, they have few people to discuss this with, and they may not even have the words and confidence to explore their real feelings. They may be reluctant to reveal how vulnerable they feel.

Lori, 49, is an exception. She says, "I'm not happy about aging, losing my health, sexuality taking on a different form, etc. But finally, I am coming out the other end of this struggle. The forties to me were all about developing new skills, coming to terms with the aging process, and finding a new physical style that projects what I am about these days: still sexy, still a vibrant woman, but less and less concerned with the good opinion of others. The last couple of years have been a grieving process for me. Saying goodbye to the old me. But now, I am so excited about what I am going to accomplish in the next 20, 30, or 40 years."

In their forties, most women want help with the emotional changes of perimenopause that keep them feeling off balance. Marlene, Louise, and Julia have all struggled with their physical and emotional balance. In comparison, Kathy has been relatively unaffected. Although it's easy to think that things should happen just like they did for a relative or friend, that's not the case. Forties Women often feel their emotions are completely out of control, and to make matters worse, they see the spreading impact on family and friends. Most women ask, "How can I control this? Is what I'm feeling normal?"

When Sarah entered perimenopause at age 43, she became so depressed that her successful freelance writing business shrank down to writing low-paying articles and conducting telephone interviews for a local business journal. She could not bring herself to reach out for other work. Her mother had died a few years before, her best friend had left town, and her husband didn't know how to help, so she simply endured. In fact, she didn't even realize she had been depressed until years later when she looked back. If she had just been able to connect with other women to compare notes and share feelings, instead of sitting alone at her desk, she might have saved herself a lot of pain.

We've heard many women say, "There is depression in my family, so I'll probably get it." Although there may be a familial component, depression is never normal. A woman needs to see her doctor because there are so many excellent treatments.

Severe clinical depression is not the same thing as occasionally feeling a little blue. Most women experience mild depression or the blues now and then, and these may respond to herbal remedies and behavioral measures including exercise and counseling. However, severe clinical depression requires medication.

Everyone gets the blues now and then, but ongoing depression is neither normal nor inevitable. Women can find the medical and psychological help needed to feel good about themselves and enjoy their life. The hormonal fluctuations of perimenopause can take emotions on a roller coaster ride similar to that of adolescence. Anxiety and the blues can develop and a woman's fears of losing beauty and energy can escalate into fears of losing her mind. Some women begin to experience full-blown anxiety attacks for the first time.

It's critically important that women find healthcare providers and support systems to guide them if they are having a painful or difficult transition. Women often suffer needlessly because they do not tell their doctors about their health concerns. In fact, many women feel that their healthcare providers don't listen well and don't seem to care much about them as patients once they have passed their childbearing years. Perhaps they remain silent because they expect no more help than Julia received, or they may allow inertia and insurance concerns to trap them in an unsatisfactory professional relationship.

Often women take great care of others but deny and ignore their true health risks. Although many women say they worry about their health, few of them can identify a specific health concern. Women need to get their own health off that back burner and generate the energy to take care of themselves before they develop a serious illness.

Health education campaigns of recent years have been taking effect. A decade ago fewer than one-third of women realized that heart disease is the number one killer of women. Today that number has risen to nearly half. Deaths from heart disease have been dropping for years. That's great news. Doctors tell us the majority of chronic and disabling illnesses are tied to lifestyle choices that we can change. That's the most important message here: We can change.

For most women, the concerns of aging go beyond their looks to a general loss of vitality and energy. I'm happy to report women can do lots of things to improve the way they feel. It's no secret. Once we get started, we love it and never want to go back. These can be the greatest and most energetic years of our lives, especially if we find a form of exercise we enjoy, perhaps even with a friend. Eating lots of fruits and vegetables, and minimizing sugar and white flour, helps stabilize weight and helps a woman feel much better. Women who rarely let themselves get eight hours of sleep a night need to cross things off their to-do lists to create space for adequate rest. Everyone has a restless night now and then, but women who usually don't rest well because of worry about the past or the future need to get professional help. It's no different than having an infected toe and every woman deserves to feel rested.

MIRROR, MIRROR, ON THE WALL

Most women have issues about their appearance and many struggle with their self-image. The Earth Mother who is committed to "natural" values like yoga and health foods strives for clear, make-up-free skin and relishes her long, flowing hair (oh, lucky genetic inheritance). Even so, she has an investment in her looks. So also the Spa Queen who, lacking the Earth Mother's genetics, pursues her desired look by spending big bucks at her hairdresser, nail technician, personal trainer and, eventually, plastic surgeon.

Each of these women cares about her self-image, but in different ways. They may even be friends. The Spa Queen may envy the effortless look of the natural beauty (although she would not dream of imitating it). The Earth Mother may vehemently reject the choices of nip and tuck, dye and perm. Yet, she knows her Spa Queen friend is not a shallow person. Rather than criticize her friend, she rejects the values of the larger beauty culture. Let's face it: despite their different paths they are both kindred souls seeking peace and acceptance of their self-images. Although they handle their changing appearance differently, both want the opportunity to see what life brings them.

Forties Women have to come to terms both with their changing self-images and society's changing views of them. Most feel ambivalent about growing older. In some ways they may feel better than ever. They are physically and emotionally strong and proud of their experiences and accomplishments. They can take a compliment without blushing or negating the statement. Some, like Louise, are ready to speak out and let the world hear them roar. Yet at the same time they can feel invisible, unheard, and dismissed by younger as well as older colleagues. Older women may feel pushed to the back row when they are in situations where pretty, amiable, or outrageous younger women get all the attention. "Not fair," is a common cry from women who have not yet created another foundation for their self-esteem.

Although many women shrug off the physical changes of wrinkles, loss of muscle tone, graying hair, and weight gain, others feel confused and frustrated. All of them speak scathingly about the media's reinforcement of today's beauty culture. Women universally resent the society that disrespects the life experiences that have earned them "black belts" in living and focuses instead on their fading looks and loss of youth.

. . . .

Sitting in an important meeting I touched my face and found my first chin hair. I tried to act as if nothing had happened but I struggled to get a grip.

. . . .

Why do women compare themselves to others? It's a common female characteristic that begins in grade school and often centers on weight. This can get worse around age 40, when metabolism slows and hormonal changes contribute to weight gain. Of course, this is all about perception; it's in our minds. A woman who feels pretty good about herself may notice those who are fatter; a woman who feels insecure may notice mostly those who are thinner. Although she may not be able to choose what she notices, she can at least work on her self-talk. She can look past the surface in herself and in others and notice the fullness of her life and world.

When women seem frozen in time they cannot imagine themselves as old and may make increasingly strenuous efforts to fit into the youth culture. This makes them easy targets for professional marketers of beauty products like the tooth whitening strips purported to let us "Lose 10 years in 7 days" or "Use this product for seven days and lose 10 years." (Where do those 10 years go? I've always wondered.)

Mothers: what are your daughters learning about aging from you?

Speaking of easy targets, women often succumb and spend too much on a product and then felt bad about it. In reality, they need to lighten up and take it easy on themselves. Laugh about it! After all, good skin care and good self-care just makes sense.

More women say their attitudes toward aging resemble those of their mothers than do not. The bond with her mother is the first, strongest relationship every girl encounters. Mothers exert a powerful influence, primarily by their actions. Although we may hear their words, we model our behavior and attitudes primarily on what we see them do.

Although many women admit to seeing more and more of their mother in themselves as they grow older, women in their forties are still eager to point out ways they differ from their moms: "I'm more vain." "I'm more successful." "I'm living out her dream." "I have different attitudes."

With role models like Julia's mom, it's no wonder so many women stifle their questions and concerns and suffer in silence. Julia and Louise, who believe that loneliness is associated with aging, reflect their experiences with models who viewed aging as a fearful time of loss. In contrast, Kathy and Marlene, who do not perceive their mothers as struggling with aging, view it more as a rite of passage filled with experience, knowledge, and respect for the older woman.

The question, "Mothers: what are your daughters learning about aging from you?" is worth asking. Knowing that a daughter was watching and learning by example has spurred many women to change. I sought ongoing education and ultimately a doctorate in clinical psychology in large part because I wanted to show my three daughters that they could do anything they wanted. Another friend found the courage to leave an abusive husband when she realized that by staying, she was teaching her nine-year-old daughter that such a relationship was acceptable.

Without positive role models women may opt for repeated surgeries like Julia's mother did. One pitfall is that they can begin to look like brittle porcelain dolls after repeated procedures. What will your young daughter do when she reaches your age? Will she find peace, joy, and acceptance in her later years? Or will she feel guilt and dismay when she loses her youthful glow, afraid that she has somehow failed to do enough to keep it, buy it, or want it bad enough to stay young and beautiful?

Forties Women are working hard to refine their personal style to reflect the new person they are becoming. They are looking in the mirror, looking behind at their youth and looking at the years ahead, trying to make sense of their aging experience. They may try on activities and attitudes like a pair of new shoes. "Does this fit the occasion? Does this feel good? Is it me?"

This "trying on for size" occurs in concrete fashion challenges as well. Louise worries about being judged for wearing short skirts, but the paradox is that women may receive criticism from someone — usually another woman — regardless of what they choose. Someone will criticize them if they dress like younger women or if they choose clothing that is more "age appropriate," whatever that means. There are no written guidelines or manuals on how become "an older woman." If she lets her hair turn gray, some women will say she has given up; if she dyes her hair and dresses in the latest styles, some will complain she is trying to fool Mother Nature. Can the older woman win? The best place to find help and support is from her women friends.

IT HURTS: SURVIVING LOVE AND LOSS

Some of the most unnerving changes of midlife occur when roles and relationships shift among family and friends. Children become more independent and even leave home. Marriages hit the 20-year mark and may start to feel stale. Their nests start to empty and they grieve a variety of losses. Still, these familial changes are not a major source of aging anxiety for most Forties Women.

Loss of a primary intimate relationship affects attitudes toward getting older, although not in any expected way. Women who are married, widowed, or divorced fear aging at a much lower rate than women who are separated or women who have never married. Marlene, divorced, is not afraid. Julia, never married, is afraid. Perhaps the unresolved aspect of separation or singleness triggers aging anxiety. Women seem to know that their health and well-being is better when they have strong ties to others, and aging seems to be less bothersome for those with strong support systems of friends and family, a deep spiritual life, and strong ties within the community.

Those who are most successful usually seize this time of change as an opportunity to re-define themselves. Our parents begin to need our support more than they provide it. Learning to see them as frail humans can help us let go of old angers and resentments. Kathy feels stuck between two roles as her children become more self-sufficient. In fact, they are offering support to her by researching new possibilities for her to pursue. Such role reversals may help women like Louise who are interested in re-careering to find a new field that interests them. By example, we in turn can teach our children to be aware of reinvention in a world of possibilities.

One of the most painful realities of aging, women say, is the sense that they are losing societal support they enjoyed when they were younger. Many report feeling disregarded and even "invisible." June, a 47-year-old lesbian retail shop owner, says scornfully, "Feeling invisible is usually just about losing the attention of men." Other women feel it goes deeper and broader than that: a lack of respect and regard can be conveyed by younger women, store clerks, and even family members who discount an older woman's opinions.

"It annoys me when I'm with my co-workers, and I might as well not be in the room," Louise says. "I don't get the same nods, eye contact, or acceptance of my ideas that I once did. I've never asked other women if they have similar problems, because I'm afraid it's just me." There is not much a woman can do to change the attitudes of people around her, and if her work environment becomes too negative, she should develop an escape plan. Many women start their own businesses. At the very least, a woman should ensure that she has areas in her life in which she feels effective, heard, and valued.

THE SMART, GOOD-LOOKING FORTIES

The forties are a confusing time full of surprises, challenges, emotions, and promises. Even strong women like Louise, who has opinions and is not afraid to share them, may question their futures in the bedroom and in the world. Many Forties Women use the newly available time, freed up from childrearing, to build upon successful relationships, often deepening them into close, trusting friendships. Partners are becoming comfortable companions. Some women say they want to be closer and rekindle the romance they once had with their husbands. Others want a partner who will walk with them and allow them to continue their personal and professional growth. For still others, Mr. Right has shown up at last.

"At 49, my body is changing, and men my age are changing, too," Lori noted. "We're not as flexible as before." The best relationships change as each partner changes and both parties accept and support this process.

By forty, most women have accepted that their spouses won't fill all their needs and they are investing in other relationships, notably with women friends and community activities. Some are returning to the workplace and others are considering it for the first time. When she begins searching for a new role in life, the Forties Woman may have to learn anew how to put herself first. She has often lost touch with what she enjoys or would want, not for her kids or for the community, but for herself. "If this were my life," she should ask herself, "What would I want to do?"

There are so many advantages to getting older that a woman could easily focus her full attention on the pluses. Rediscovering romance with someone she truly knows and deeply trusts. The arrival of grandchildren she can adore and spoil. Using newfound time for herself to expand her circle of friends. Finding and becoming a role model and mentor.

If we expect to continue to be interesting to others, we must be interested in them and in our wider world. Think of the timeless women you know. Do they sit at home crying and waiting for life to come to them? Do they hide their fears of aging and act as if they couldn't care less, but in the dark of night search their computer or watch infomercials in search of a magic anti-aging potion? Not likely. Women like Kathy and Marlene reject such superficial solutions and take matters into their own hands. They look to their friends, mentors, and role models to help them develop their plans and prepare themselves for life's inevitable changes.

But not everyone is fortunate enough to have a supportive circle of women friends and many feel insecure about reaching out to find a mentor. So where can you find support? Seize your right to openly discuss your fears of aging rather than burying them under the futile attempt to stay looking young.

FORTIES WOMEN WANT OTHERS TO KNOW

. . . .

- ❧ I am worried that my time to be who I really want to be is running out.
- ❧ I am often torn between what I want and what others want from me.
- ❧ I want to have passion and purpose in my life but I'm too overloaded to figure out what that might be.
- ❧ I feel guilty when I yearn to say, "I want time just for me."
- ❧ I want my partner to see me as an exciting and passionate woman and still be attracted to me.
- ❧ I worry more about my looks when I see the physical changes in my face and body.

see sidebar next page

Where can a woman find support? After participating in a 12-step program, Suzanne, 48, finally accepted that her birth brothers were never going to care about her the way she wanted. Only half joking, she asked, "Am I too old to be adopted?" In time, though, she realized she could — and did — ask two dear family friends if they would become her brothers. They agreed, and now they always share special hugs and affection at social gatherings, and occasionally meet for lunch. One of the best consequences is that Suzanne has been able to let go of her anger and disappointment with her birth family. This approach could help Julia deal with her feeling of lack in her relationship with her mother.

Change continues to occur through the forties and many women say they steadily gain confidence they could not have imagined earlier. They become more willing to risk, to step out of their comfort zone, and to try new things. Look around at work, at church, in the community, even in the family. Kathy found mentors and friends everywhere. It's second nature to her now, but women can start by identifying people they admire for anything. The next step is to think of what might be offered in return, from gratitude to babysitting to landscaping to a great cookie recipe. Then it's time to reach out. (This is the part where they allow themselves to feel a little or a lot uncomfortable.) They can gather their courage and ask if they might call for a little advice on that issue, or meet for coffee. Most people are flattered to be asked and love to help. If a woman encounters someone who declines, she should know the refusal probably is nothing personal, and try again.

Letting one's light shine outward is a great way to get connected. Every woman has something to offer and should consider becoming a mentor to others. Worrying what others will think may keep a woman from reaching out to others. At all times, a woman should be gentle with herself, and if this is all just too difficult, should consider getting professional help. Every woman deserves to feel strong and supported.

Do women worry about getting older because of what men will think? Not usually. Far more often, women say that attitudes towards aging are influenced by society, culture, and other women than by men's ideas. Research into today's beauty culture reveals women's appearance worries center on the judgment of other women. Women's ability to influence each other highlights the importance of becoming a role model or mentor. It also points out the importance of choosing her friends carefully. If she feels terribly pressured about her appearance, she should get rid of her mirrors and seek out people who focus on deeper values.

Menopause is a major life transition; as such, it is a wake-up call and a time for reassessment. Women should ask, "Am I where I want to be with my health, relationships, career, and financial situation?" Most women in their forties are supremely confident of their ability to care for themselves. They see themselves as vital and active; they set goals for themselves that are as high — or higher — than when they were 20 and 30 years old. They continue to expect themselves to either realize or re-evaluate goals like pursuing a dream, returning to a career, or choosing a new career.

FORTIES WOMEN WANT OTHERS TO KNOW

- ❀ I find my emotions get the best of me and leave me confused and eager to just relax.

- ❀ I worry about not having enough energy to do all the things I have to do.

- ❀ My drive and motivations are changing and I want to be first and not in second or last place.

Many women in their forties have achieved career advancement, been recognized for their talent, found joy in mothering older and younger children, or have discovered the benefits of a single life. Nonetheless, money emerges consistently as a top concern for every age group and caring for self blends into this concern.

Although money is a major concern for women in their forties, they rarely talk about their concerns. It's as if many of them feel unable to affect that area of their lives. Women who work in positions that are traditionally paid less than men, and who have less authority than the men around them, may feel powerless. Many women in their forties have watched their mothers struggle with finances, or have gone through painful divorces, or believe their pay scale will never catch up to that of their male co-workers. None of this has to happen. Every woman can seize her power and take control of her work life. Gain new skills to earn more and overhaul your budget to spend less. Adopt one new healthy habit each month. Speak honestly and take responsibility for your feelings. You have the power to change your life.

Improve Your Job Performance

- Get employer expectations in writing.
- Ask for feedback between performance evaluations.
- Document your performance.
- Ask for evaluations and disciplinary actions in writing.
- Take criticism seriously.
- Work to correct problems.

Earn More Money

- Ask for specifics on pay ranges.
- Ask around to learn pay ranges in your market.
- Ask how you can be more valuable to your organization.
- Ask for specifics on what you should be doing to earn pay increases.

Advance Your Career

- Be willing to learn new skills.
- Take on new assignments.
- Do the extra 10 percent.
- Upgrade your knowledge of your industry through training.
- Take advantage of tuition reimbursement programs.
- Monitor how you conduct yourself with supervisors and colleagues outside your job.
- Don't gossip, complain, or exert negative influence.
- Avoid habitual tardiness or taking too much sick time.

The life questions women ask are important ones and not to be taken lightly. "Who will care for me? Can I afford health care? How long will I have to work? How long will I be able to work? Can I ever afford to retire? Will I have the money to pay my bills now and until I die?" One thing is certain. If a woman in her forties has not learned to plan financially for her future, it is high time she started learning to manage her own affairs. Women in their forties can easily live forty more years, so they must learn to take a more active role in earning, financial planning, and managing their affairs. She should educate herself, join an investment club, find a mentor. Time is still on her side as she works to accumulate the cash to fund her old age.

Earning power aside, what back-burner issues, projects, goals, and dreams need to come forward as a woman heads into the second half of life?

LIVE THE LIFE YOU WANT

- Help others help you through networking and mentorships.
- Don't ally yourself too closely with one supervisor or mentor.
- Know what you want.
- Learn your strengths and maximize them.
- Learn your weaknesses and minimize them.
- Set priorities for your life and career.
- Be flexible and open to new opportunities.
- Prepare to be lucky.

Long-suppressed personal needs may clamor for attention. Might these interests provide a springboard for a new career?

The forties are a time many women undertake a whole-person check. Many are beginning to understand for the first time that their aging process is real, and that it is time to consider their options and begin developing an action plan. Whose responsibility is it if one is not happy?

One of the most wonderful things about the forties is that women begin to reawaken to their own interests. Single women often have a head start on learning to put themselves first, but by now most women are looking inward for their power and reawakening to their own talents. They dust off goals and desires they had set aside during their childrearing years, and now begin to relish their new freedom.

It's good news to see that as we get older, we make progress with our fears. Although many women are becoming a little more willing to talk to each other about their fears and concerns, others allow their fears to isolate them. For every woman who takes aging in stride and draws comfort from a solid support group, nearly as many struggle with their fears, feeling lost and alone.

Women are more likely to struggle with aging when they equate their inevitable loss of beauty and youth with a loss of value and desirability. They may feel alone with few social resources and little support, which makes the universe a pretty unfriendly place. The absence of successful female role models can leave them obsessing about not being able to care for themselves when they are old. They often have multiple health issues that they feel unable to correct and they sit silently and bear the burden of their fears alone.

Without contact with friends, women have no one with whom they might share their concerns and gain reassurance about normal reactions to aging. We must help each other find ways to cope with these fears because aging, after all, is normal and the single inevitable, unavoidable alternative to dying. It's part of the cycle of life.

Women are more likely to age successfully when they plan for their futures and do not sit passively by and let the world dictate their fate. When they see aging as a natural process that they can influence through their own efforts they are more likely to maintain good health and good relationships and stay connected with their worlds. Instead of dwelling on things they cannot change or spending time glued to the mirror looking for youth and beauty, they find their purpose and passion and set out to make a difference in this world. When they can find their satisfaction and support with new and challenging people, places, and activities they are more likely to understand that the source of love and happiness is within themselves. Women who have learned from positive role models how to grow older happily often stay positive and find comfort in their faith that their lives are unfolding as they should.

Dr. Nancy's Kick-Butt Keys for Forties Women

- Bring your attention into your present reality. Release fears and losses from the past or future to increase your ability to impact your real life.
- Counteract fear by sending out love for yourself and others; allow your inner light to shine out.
- Discuss your fears with someone you trust and seek healing laughter about the human condition.
- Investigate your spirituality through organized religion or other faith. Many people say faith removes fear.
- Get busy. Is there anyone in your world who has bigger problems than you do? Can you help?
- Heed your fear. Are you worried about money? Health? Relationships? Maybe you should be. Take responsibility for making improvements.
- Dare. Bravely take baby steps into areas that make you uncomfortable. Find a trusted companion or guide to give you feedback. Take risks. Embrace your life.
- One of your most valuable resources is contact with other people. To find them, revisit your personal interests and goals and start doing things you enjoy.
- Watch community announcements in the paper, library, online, or church. Join an organization and volunteer for a committee. Become involved.
- Invite members of the group to other activities: lunch, a movie, a walk. Take an interest in others. Ask about their lives and remember what they say.

On the whole, Forties Women feel they have come a long way. Like Marlene, they have learned a lot about taking care of themselves. Sure, they cannot be certain what lies ahead, and they sometimes feel scared about the external changes that appear without warning. All in all, however, they like what they have learned about who they are, and they don't feel they have changed all that much on the inside when it comes to feeling young.

. . . .

I say a prayer
and try not to dwell
on the negative.

. . . .

By the time they leave their forties, women feel secure in their places as valued members of their communities. They are making peace with the women they have become and are finding ways to love and respect themselves at last. "Now, I'll meet with people about anything as long as it's not a confrontation," says Julia. "I know how to pick my battles. The sooner a woman gets self-confidence and the ability to say, 'This is who I am and what I stand for,' the easier her life will be."

Now, let's see what women say about the Big Five-Oh.

Visit www.womenspeak.com to learn more about the forties. Express yourself and share ways you have learned, grown, and found your best life.

CHAPTER 5   *The* *50s*
Finding Philosophy — Me,
or God or What?

I am having a ball now that I've learned to say no to them
and yes to me!

JUNE, 53

In her sixth decade, a Fifties Woman realizes that she is more than halfway through her ride. A woman who celebrates her fifty-first birthday today can expect to live at least another 31 years to become 82. Many will live much longer. The years are picking up speed, and she has learned to squeeze more life out of every minute. This acceleration leads women to cultivate their personal philosophies of life. Some women move toward acceptance of time's passing, while others are in denial. Every Fifties Woman comments that the way she feels inside no longer matches the image she sees in the mirror.

Still filled with vibrancy and vitality, members of this Baby Boomer generation flatly refuse to feel old and are determined to reinvent themselves. They have been called The Great Postponers because they do not like to consider themselves as aging, and they have rejected the label "middle-aged."

WHAT FIFTIES WOMEN WORRY ABOUT

The Fifties Woman faces a host of new changes and challenges. Menopause is a reality for nearly everyone before this decade is over, and changing sexuality bring up questions of identity. Financial questions come to the fore. As the far-off prospect of retirement inches closer, she thinks more often about her future security and her desire and ability to continue working. This is complicated by the fact that she may begin to feel age discrimination in the workplace and face competition from workers much younger than herself. The empty nest of many

Fifties Women may refill with divorced children and grandchildren and they may find themselves sandwiched between the demands of aging parents, children, and grandchildren.

Fifties Women feel especially successful about getting older when they shift their focus from caring for others and begin to improve the care they take of themselves. The changing focus of activities can lead to adjustments in relationships as well. For most, their psychological health is good and many are newly determined to work harder on their physical health. And despite the emotional pain of divorce, many find that the end of an unsatisfactory marriage actually provides a new and exciting beginning.

Fifties Women experience a wide range of feelings, not the least of which is relief. They are into letting go of the past and reinventing themselves in this new phase of life. Delighted to be able at last to take a deep breath when children are raised, many say, "This is *my* time!" They become especially interested in reaching out in friendship to other women as they have gained confidence to say to family members, "You're on your own for dinner tonight, I'm going out with the girls."

In this chapter we meet Sarah, Ruth, Betsey, and Jane; each woman has developed her own unique style for retaining her youthful verve at the half-century mark. The fifties are a wonderful time of renewed freedom and opportunity for women. They stretch out of their earlier roles and look around with confidence, asking "What now?"

SARAH: "STAYING IN THE MOMENT HELPS ME LIVE SUCCESSFULLY."

Sarah is 55 and married, a former marketing executive who recently changed careers. "I worked primarily with younger girls who were like my children in a lot of respects. I was at a loss to find someone my age to talk to, someone who understood hot flashes and senior moments. They hadn't experienced life yet like I have and their interests were different than mine." Sarah felt weird, stuck between youth and old age. "I felt like I didn't fit."

She had always done lots of volunteer work in her children's schools. When the school district's foundation executive left, Sarah worked for weeks to recruit a new person to fill this important position. Suddenly she thought, "Why don't I think that I can do this?" So she applied and she got the job. The new challenge has energized her work life, and she expects to work until age 70 — or beyond. The image of a leisurely retirement in a Sun City environment holds no appeal for her whatsoever.

She does not fear her own aging process and tries each day to count her blessings. As far as Sarah is concerned, aging is a normal process. "It's just the evolution of a woman's life, not a disease. It's not even a problem although it is good for women to talk together about our issues. Together we can look at natural health solutions and share our experiences.

"Remember that today, at this moment in your life, you cannot change what happened yesterday, nor can you change what will happen tomorrow," says Sarah. "Staying in the moment is what will help me to live successfully as I get older."

Sarah is a confirmed feminist who favors equal opportunity and equal pay for equal work. This doesn't mean she believes that boys and girls are the same. "I raised my kids as much as possible without gender bias," she recalls. "I gave my daughter a toolbox and toy truck, and gave my son dishes and a doll. My daughter quickly used the truck as a stepstool so she could get up on the counter to reach my jewelry and makeup. She used the toolbox as a dish drainer. My son used the dishes as Frisbees and the doll was quickly reduced to its component parts. A lot of gender differences are simply genetic. But that doesn't mean women should earn less for the same work."

After 22 years of marriage, her younger child is in high school and her nest is nearly empty, which leaves her and her husband dealing directly with each other again. "My husband and I are rediscovering what life was like 20 years ago," Sarah says. "It's good. My life with him hasn't been all hearts and flowers, but we have arrived at a calm appreciation of each other that is quite comforting."

Feeling her body change, Sarah wishes she felt more comfortable talking about her sexuality. "Sometimes I wonder if he still finds me all that attractive after all these years." She misses the sexy old days, yet has not been able to mention to her doctor how uncomfortable sex has become. She wonders what is wrong with her and frets because her husband is disappointed in her waning desire.

Sarah has been feeling the approach of menopause, and her hot flashes keep her from getting a good night's sleep. "I thought there was something wrong until I talked with my sister. She said that getting up at three A.M. to sleep on the couch was so common. Who knew? I'm not crazy after all!"

She continually checks her rear view in the mirror and says with chagrin, "I just hate my sagging butt. No stretch pants for me any more." She wonders why she has not taken better care of herself, and whether she has the energy to start exercising more. And no matter how hard she exercises she knows in her heart that buns of steel will elude her. Last week she picked up some green tea supplements because a friend told her this would rev up her energy and her system and the pounds would melt off. She laughs at herself, though, saying, "This is where it all starts, the quest for the perfect antidote to Mother Nature's calling card, better known as gravity."

Sarah thinks that weighing less and aging without wrinkles would be a nice plus, but she's realistic about the likelihood. She's not willing to change her eating habits and she knows that wrinkles run in her family. Her main wish for her future is really to maintain her strength and independence and not be a burden to others. If she could change something about the world, she would build a stronger role for older women in our society and make better use of them as important resources for generations coming along behind.

"I think women do age more successfully than men because we handle life crises and survive change better than men. We're more resilient, probably because women are more realistic about the present and the future." Sarah has always looked to her women friends to help her through life much more than her husband. They talk on the phone regularly, get together to dance, eat and talk, talk, talk. "It's our sisterhood," she says.

Growing up with Depression-era parents, Sarah and her birth sisters learned a lot about fear. "Some of my sisters are so tight-fisted, they'll never give themselves anything new or good," she says. "They're all, 'Oh, I'll take the burnt toast,' and 'No, you take the biggest piece.'"

Sarah is different. Although she won't go into debt for material things, if she has money, she's not afraid to spend it. "Many women think 'I'll take time for myself later' but it's never later. All we have is today."

Her mother was diagnosed with breast cancer in her early fifties, so Sarah is highly motivated to practice prevention. She had a skin cancer removed at age fifty — no big deal, quick recovery. But the doctor said it's likely to recur. It's always in the back of my mind."

Still, Sarah doesn't worry much about getting sick. What's much more important to her is to know that she is living life, that she has survived. Beyond doing her best for her health, she believes worry is pointless. "We either die or get better. Either way it resolves itself eventually."

"Human life isn't very long," she says. "But we and our children and our grandchildren are all connected. There's a higher power outside of ourselves. In life I have seen that when one door closes, another opens. Dying is just another door."

· ·

SARAH ISN'T AFRAID OF GETTING older and she relishes the fact that she has been married a long time. She and her husband are doing well to take this opportunity to rediscover their strengths and the basis of their marriage. There's nothing about a long marriage that is easy, and they are focusing on the good and building on it.

Even women who have a close circle of friends often worry alone about their aging sexual anatomy. Women traditionally feel such a deep reserve talking about their sexual lives that the subject may never come up, even within groups of very close, long-time friends. Even if they can't bring themselves to talk with their friends, Fifties Women can easily find help for their vaginal distress by leveling with a gynecologist. Hormonal changes cause what doctors call genital atrophy; the fix is topical hormones from various sources that can restore those tissues to health.

Sarah has always avoided mainstream medicine in favor of alternative approaches, which has served her well in the past. Although there have been no large studies on the so-called bioidentical hormones offered by compounding pharmacies, some women who use these pharmaceutical products are pleased with their results. Whatever she decides to do, Sarah owes it to herself and her relationship to get help with this issue. If her alternative methods do not provide her with the relief she needs, I hope she will not give up but instead will give traditional healthcare a chance to help. Aside from worrying about her weight (which she could control with a few changes in her diet and exercise patterns) Sarah feels she has done pretty well by her health. She is reaping the benefits of her healthy lifestyle and feels strong and powerful.

Women born of Depression-era parents often do well in mapping out their own financial strategies and priorities. They saw many role models in their parents' generation who sacrificed their own gratification and satisfaction to benefit others, so they must work hard to believe in themselves as worthy of investment and effort. Sarah and her husband have handled their money worries together and learned communication skills that enable them to make good decisions.

Faith often takes a larger role in Fifties Women's lives as well, and this helps them deal with uncertainties of the future. With one last child nearly ready to leave home, Sarah is looking forward to her empty nest and wants to seize every opportunity to have fun with her husband in this last half of her life.

RUTH: "NEVER LET THEM KNOW YOUR AGE."

In contrast to Sarah, Ruth is dreading turning 58 on her next birthday. Her biggest worry is becoming "invisible" to her co-workers. As a professional stockbroker, her job requires her to look good, perform well, and compete with other money managers rising through the ranks, both male and female, many of whom are much younger than she.

"I think it's important to look as good as I can, so I buy good cosmetics and try to take care of my skin," she says. Although she suspects it's an illusion, she still occasionally buys new products she sees on television that promise to minimize her wrinkles and make her look 10 years younger.

She worries so much about keeping up that she is considering having a face-lift. "If that's what it takes to compete, I'll do it," she says. Ruth worries about what other women and men will think of her, so much so that she even consulted a professional career consultant and takes to heart his advice: "Never let them know your age and never talk about hot flashes. It will only age you in the eyes of your co-workers and reduce your marketability."

The other girls at work are younger, mostly married with kids. "After 20 years in my brokerage house, I'm the oldest woman at work. The men are looked up to. Although the men will come and ask me things, the girls tend to go to the men." Lately she has been seeking out women her own age to find someone she can relate to and asks, "Do you ever feel like this?"

She loves keeping busy with her job and draws tremendous satisfaction from being a high-earner. "I honestly don't think I'll ever retire," Ruth says, "because I can't imagine stopping doing something that I love. And I refuse to be forced out."

Ruth believes that her Thirties Women co-workers neglect their health. "They won't do breast self-exams or screenings, not even a girl whose mom died of breast cancer. Men physicians often say young women don't need mammograms, but thousands of women in their twenties and thirties are being diagnosed with breast cancer every year, often in a much later stage than older women. I worry they don't look out for themselves."

She also worries about their financial well-being. Many of her younger co-workers think they have to buy name-brand products for their kids. "They get so far in debt, they'll refinance their house and max their credit cards. They can't see what they're doing to their futures."

Ruth knows how a bleak future feels. "I lived with one man my entire life," she confides. "He was alcoholic and abusive, and for years my 12-step program is what kept me going. We're still in that generation where men are dominant. We live with the double standard. I'm the granddaughter of an old-fashioned Baptist preacher. My standards were that I couldn't have sex before marriage, so I married as a teen for lust, not for love. Then I stuck with it because I had married 'forever.' He got the better and I got the worse.

"I was the codependent wife of an alcoholic and my life was a mess at home, but I worked in the business world to get respect. I lived two lives for many years and they never met," she says. "I finally got him to go with me to a counselor. My husband was so skilled at manipulating me that *I* appeared the one with the anger problem when he was actually the rageaholic. I called a friend who said 'Quit the counseling, quit the Al-Anon. Go back to what you had before because he's going to build a case against you and you'll lose your kids.'"

At age 52, Ruth took her three sons and daughter and divorced her husband of 24 years. "I finally woke up to the fact that I'm worth something. There's something golden inside of me that flickers, and the only thing I have to give my children is *me*. This book is important because the wisdom of women has never been recorded and I want that for my daughter. Now I have a bounce in my walk and I don't have to hide a thing, including my laugh lines!"

After her children grew up and moved out, she found she missed them tremendously, especially her daughter. "Even though I hadn't doted on her — I mean, I didn't cry when she got her period, or anything like that — still it bothered me when she left."

By Ruth's choice, her daughter moved back in with her own kids while pursuing a bachelor of nursing degree at age 40. "She could have done it other ways but this was easier, and I liked our combination of four women in three generations. But I'm ready for my nest to be empty again."

Although she divorced her husband five years ago, she hadn't been able to free herself from the hold he had on her, despite the fact that he had actually passed away. "Then about a month ago, I had a dream that I finally — literally and physically — pushed him out of my life. I took my power back, which makes me wonder why I ever let it get away in the first place! One week later I met a wonderful new man. On our first date he said, 'I had a beautiful marriage and would like to marry again.' I said 'That's nice, I had a terrible marriage and doubt I'll *ever* marry again.' I'm not certain I could do all the compromises. We went through so much unhappiness at home, I always figured no one would be good enough for me or my kids." When Ruth hears stories about a happy marriage and people comfortably growing old together, she feels angry that she never had it. "But maybe now with this new man I see a possibility of having that sense of comfort and ease with someone."

With this new relationship, Ruth has discovered a renewed interest in sex. "It's a much more important part of my life now, although I still have a hard time talking about it. I would like to know if what I'm going through is normal—what do others experience? But I don't know how to bring it up."

"If only I could erase my past health sins," she says. "I smoked and spent a lot of time broiling in the sun. I go to the dermatologist regularly, and nothing has developed yet. But I do worry about melanoma and other types of skin cancer." She's proud of herself for quitting smoking, but hates the weight she gained in the process. That gives her another worry: will excess pounds hurt her health? "It's weird, I've been worrying about dying, which I have never thought about before," she says. "Maybe it's just an age thing."

She also wishes she had saved more money when she was younger and had planned better as she grew older. Despite her high earnings, her husband spent everything so she has little put away for her future, a situation she recognizes in so many women she works with at the brokerage. "Many women suddenly find themselves alone," she says. "Their husband either dies or leaves them for a younger woman. Suddenly you are on your own. It's important to prepare yourself emotionally, physically, and financially for the single life."

Ruth loves working and sees her growing backlog of experiences as helpful. "Although I guess my age does limit some of my relationships at work, I think I have a youthful attitude that helps my younger co-workers feel comfortable."

Despite what the consultant told her about hiding her age, and setting aside her own fears of aging, Ruth is feeling freer as she gets older to do what she wants much more often than before. She also is *much* less concerned about what others think of her behavior. "I give myself more permission each day to say and do the things I really want, and without spending the rest of the day worrying if I made a fool of myself. Age really does have its privileges."

. . . .

ALTHOUGH RUTH IS DELIGHTED TO have at last divorced her abusive husband, and is pleased with her steadily increasing earning power, in her heart she is still apprehensive about getting older. Pressure to compete in her workplace has increased her fears of becoming invisible and irrelevant in her brokerage firm, and she is seeking cosmetic tools to improve her standing.

Ruth's largest area of concern is her career. Fifties Women often feel pressure in the workplace due to other people's beliefs about age. Because of those misconceptions, they feel ignored, like they are becoming invisible. Although a few Forties Women mentioned this concern, the complaint becomes much more common in the fifties age cohort.

Although Ruth is delighted with the budding relationship with a new man in her life, she still says she'll never remarry. A woman who has spent agonizing years with an alcoholic may never be able to contemplate marriage with anything but revulsion. She will cherish her new feeling of freedom and relish not needing to hide who she is and how she feels. Nurturing this feeling of freedom may help a Fifties Woman like Ruth overcome her anxieties about growing older. Once she truly accepts herself, she will find that others do as well, and can get on with the business of life.

Ruth's mother was her mentor, and hung in throughout her daughter's terrible marriage without criticizing or making Ruth feel bad about herself. Having a good model who does not criticize definitely helps Fifties Women look back on their lives with forgiveness instead of condemnation. Women who feel accepted by their mothers love to open their own homes to daughters and grandchildren;

they pass along to subsequent generations a strong sense of family loyalty, flexibility, and self-acceptance.

Women who have a striking appearance in their youth enjoyed the power that came from turning heads. By the fifties, it's been a while since that happened, and Ruth has nearly gotten over grieving that loss. Although they may still occasionally worry that other women will judge their changing appearance, Fifties Women have noticed that people respond not so much to the way they look as to their level of interest in others. In fact, this is the way Ruth herself assesses new acquaintances, by their personality and friendliness.

For women like Ruth, the satisfaction of being good earners goes a long way to countering their anxieties about health and getting older. With enough additional years in the workplace and a careful savings plan, they will be able to provide for their old age and any care they may need.

As they search for new ways to think about their advancing years Fifties Women scour Web sites and bookstores looking for information. They are big consumers of self-help books and are determined to find resources to help them understand what they are going through. At this time of their lives they are working hard to feel more comfortable with the changes they are experiencing.

One common wish in this time of reassessment is that they had taken better care of themselves. They may talk a lot about becoming more active and eating better, but often have a hard time getting started. This is a perfect time for Fifties Women to build on their strengths by taking a little step each day to build new health habits. At the same time, they need to remember to be kind to themselves; they are human with weaknesses and failings.

One way women like Ruth can improve their health prospects is to schedule annual visits to a gynecologist for a Pap test, to the dermatologist for a skin check, and to regularly get a mammogram, bone density test, and colon cancer screening. Many women start to take their annual physicals more seriously when they turn 50, which is a good thing. Ruth is setting a good example for her family and friends and encourages all of them to get screened and tested each year.

BETSEY: "I DON'T HAVE MUCH OUTSIDE SUPPORT. WILL I BE ABLE TO CARRY THIS BURDEN?"

At 57, Betsey has advanced from executive secretary to office manager of a large law firm. "I can't believe how many young girls at work say, 'I'll marry and have kids and live off my husband's pension,'" she says. "I tell them, 'Don't you realize they don't even have pensions anymore? You have to take care of yourself!' Many women — especially in more rural areas — are unaware and need mentors. Women still so often don't have the guts to stand up and say No to unreasonable demands."

She is afraid of growing older. She began noticing this about 10 years ago, and she feels deeply confused about it. "I'll be feeling like I have my act together pretty well, and all of a sudden I get depressed and worry about dying," she says. In her darkest moods, she makes the macabre joke: "Maybe when we get old there will be so many of us, the Dr. Kevorkians will be taking appointments!"

Betsey has never been able to talk with anyone about these feelings and wishes she had more information about what is normal and what is out of the norm. "Most of my women friends just don't seem to have this problem with aging. They would even joke about their hot flashes." Deeply reserved, Betsey's embarrassment with the topic prevents her from talking about it with even her closest friends. Instead, she reads everything she can find in print and online to help her understand what's going on.

Competitive and optimistic, Betsey has steadily pursued her career, changing jobs as necessary to improve her prospects. She never had an interest in having children. Lately, however, she has wondered if she made a good choice and often feels acutely alone, even though she has sole responsibility for her aging mother.

Her mother just turned 80, hasn't really been doing well for several years, and can no longer live alone. Two years ago, she moved her mom into a secure facility. The first year in the Alzheimer's unit cost $70,000, far beyond her mom's Social Security and pension payments. "I don't have much outside support," Betsey says. "Will I be able to carry this burden?"

Betsey also worries about her financial security as a single woman, particularly because her own health is not that good. "I look at my mom and wonder: Will I be able to take care of myself when I am her age? I don't think I'll ever retire.

I need a reason to get up in the morning. I'm going to need money for my old age, and besides, who would I be if I'm not working?"

Over the years, Betsey has dated a lot of men, but she was happy and busy and didn't want to marry. "I thought it would be a total waste of time. I did finally agree to live with a man when I was 46 and discovered I had been right: It *was* a waste of time. He was younger than me but became disabled. It only lasted a couple years because I've got too many things to do besides babysitting."

Extricating herself from that took time and Betsey is now extremely wary of relationships. "I'm cautious now about who I let into my life. I'll share meals but I won't pick up their socks. That old adage, 'If you can get the milk for free, why buy the cow,' works both ways," she says. "A woman can have sex and companionship without a husband." Still, she is worried that men will find her too old and she does not look forward to growing old alone. Although she daydreams about having a love interest, she knows she is no longer willing to make the compromises that might be necessary to sustain a relationship.

"I have no children and no family except my mother near here, so I rely on my friends who help me through. They are my family," she says. "My fifty-second year is the year of not being the victim. I won't take shit from anybody. As I get older, I've moved to a different stage where friends are more valuable."

Betsey goes to great lengths to maintain her appearance and she hates to be around women who just "let themselves fall apart. Because I keep up my appearance, other women often feel threatened by me." She notices this especially in the social circles of men she dates, whose women friends regard Betsey with suspicion. "None of them accept me," she says. "I just concentrate on my job and the relationship, keeping my eyes on the prize. I find my women friends elsewhere."

Lately, even that security has been threatened. "So many of my friends have gotten cancer," Betsey says. "In the last six months, I found out that four women I know have breast cancer. Two are OK, one is semi-OK, one is awful. It was such a shock. I thought, 'Oh my gosh, *they are in my age group.*' One of these is a friend I work with once a year on a volunteer campaign. She's in her late fifties and works for a high-powered ad agency. She didn't want to be perceived as a feeble old lady, so she told no one. Her daughter was away living in Japan so she went through it absolutely alone. My friend made that part of herself completely invisible for fear of being judged."

With her reliance on her friends, Betsey has been a joiner. "It really helps to surround myself with positive, outgoing, and realistic women. I have a new friend in her forties and we are having a lot of fun comparing notes about growing older." They agree it's important to find someone in your life who models the older woman you would like to be, and were delighted to discover they both admired Jane Pauley. "She has gone through hard times and re-invented herself; it's really inspiring," Betsey said. Betsey's aunt is still very athletic in her seventies, loves to keep up on the latest music, and devotes her spare time to caring for what she calls "the old people."

"I wish I could accept my age more gracefully," Betsey says. "I also wish I could have done some things sooner and that I had the confidence to try new and exciting things." But, when she can push her fears aside, Betsey can say honestly, "I'm now happier than ever."

. . . .

BETSEY HAS NEVER MARRIED AND has a lot of anxieties about getting older. Her anxiety probably has a lot to do with her aging mother's attitudes and current condition. With daily responsibility to watch over her mom, Betsey has a close-up view of what her own old age may require and she is wisely paying close attention to her financial preparations.

Women like Betsey have spent their lives working on their careers rather than on a primary intimate relationship. Thanks to birth control pills, the Baby Boomer generation is the first that was able to choose to remain childless without forgoing the pleasures of sexual relationships with men. Boomer Women can devote themselves to pursuing success and getting the things that go with it.

Fifties Women who are concerned about growing older will worry about competing with younger women. Fifties men so often ignore women their own age and choose to date much younger women, in part to counteract their own worries about losing their virility. This leaves the Fifties Woman confused and wondering what is normal for a woman her age. Their great resource is the company of other women in community and professional organizations, and these connections become increasingly valuable as they reach out and explore.

Betsey feels positive on one hand and depressed on the other. When women think they are the only ones who have fears and concerns about getting older, they find it difficult to admit their worries and concerns to friends. However, if they can persist and continue to build trust, they will find they are not alone in their struggle and anger. Just talking helps them keep a sense of humor and laugh about the beauty industry's efforts to sell cosmetics, weight-loss products, and the whole concept that they should stay young and beautiful.

When she meets another woman, Betsey immediately wonders what age the other woman is and how the other woman perceives her. Women for whom age is a real issue often based their self worth on having a cute and engaging personality in their youth. When 'cute' gives way to 'mature' they resist the change and struggle to find a new identity.

Women like Betsey compare themselves to others on age, weight, dress, status, or whether or not they have the same 'beauty level.' They tend to do this with their most hated feature, or the area in which they feel least secure. Anytime Betsey enters a new group, she notices first the relative size of other women's thighs, then quickly calculates whether they are fatter or thinner than she is. This type of comparison creates a separation between women that keeps them apart and often prevents them from supporting and encouraging each other.

Looking at her own life, Betsey is determined to enjoy herself more. This is a common sentiment in Fifties Women who have tried to fulfill society's expectations (and their own) about being a devoted daughter and valuable employee. Now, having done their duty, they are ready to branch out and pursue greater satisfaction for themselves. Here again, women friends can help make the most of these opportunities.

These connections also can help a woman find resources to help fight depression and to care for ailing family members. Betsey is concerned about her own aging process, particularly her weight and her retirement funds. Money worries are never far from a Fifties Woman's consciousness, and health concerns often dominate their thinking, especially when they see friends battling serious health conditions.

Betsey is worried about growing older and at 57 she wishes to be free of her aches and pains. Fifties Women often wish their health were better, but wonder if it is too late to make changes and reverse some of their health problems. The great news is that it is most certainly not too late, and that women can see improvement and real gains within days of making lifestyle changes.

JANE: "I LOOK FORWARD TO HAVING MORE TIME FOR MY LIFE."

Jane is 55 and in great shape emotionally and physically. She recently graduated from college with a public relations degree, the oldest in her class. Shortly after delivering the commencement address she got a good job at a local hospital. Jane had delayed marriage until she was 30, had her first child at 31, and her last — the sixth — at age 40. "Watch what you pray for," she says with a laugh. "You better give God a specific number!"

Naturally, her role as a mother has shaped her life view. "Women are the creator sex," she says. "We are more open than men because we have experienced childbearing, having something growing inside of ourselves that we can't control. We have to develop trust and belief so we can carry and produce." She says the childbearing experience also introduces women to grief. "We deal early with the life-death dichotomy. Although our bodies are the incubators of new life, in the case of a miscarriage, they also become the tomb for our children."

Jane's mom died of cancer on her sixty-sixth birthday, and her father died a few years later of Alzheimer's. She found her mentors in her sixth-grade teacher and another older woman whom she visits often. "We have traveled together and they are my inspirations," she says.

Through her job, Jane became involved in a school mentoring project, which she recommends for every woman. "It is important to mentor girls, but it's equally important to mentor young men so they'll know how to respect and treat women. My daughter-in-law has commented how much she appreciates the sensitivity I instilled in my older son, but I haven't felt successful with my middle son. Through the school project I had the opportunity to mentor a young man by mediating between him and his mother," Jane says. "This was my chance to do it over and do it right. It's important to mentor as well as to learn from younger people. The world and all of us are one big global entity and it's all part of the process of being human.

. . . .

My twin bellies are a badge of courage from giving birth to twins at age 40. I have overcome my fears of having an old body.

. . . .

"My fiftieth birthday was huge for me, even though I had been too busy to think about it much. Women of all ages, whether we are very young or very old — we want respect!" Jane likes the Dove Campaign for Real Beauty that features models who are comfortable looking their age. "My crows' feet are my badge of courage," she says. "I can't regret the deepening laugh lines, because they remind me how great it felt to enjoy all those smiles and guffaws." Jane and her husband married 25 years ago. By now, all but one of their kids has moved out of the house. "I'm looking forward to having my husband all to myself," she says. "We have a ball, and it is like we are building a whole new relationship. We finally have the time to really listen to one another," Jane says. "I look forward to having more time for *my* life, and to plan our retirement and travel and our future."

Jane and her husband enjoy their lives and each other, and their love has deepened with acceptance and companionship. "We've both found a new interest in health and exercise, and we're now more active than we had ever been before. It's fun to work at building a healthy lifestyle as a couple." They feel blessed to have their family, to love their jobs, and to look forward to all the changes that life has to offer. Jane's approach to life is flexible. She knows that change is inevitable and she looks forward to new challenges.

A friend's father just died, and her mother told her they'd had sex just a week before he passed, and that it was splendid. Her dad was in his late eighties and her mom was just a few years younger. "It was more information than my friend wanted to hear, but it gave me hope that everything will still work as it should for another 30 years."

Jane overcame her fear of not being sexy by putting effort there — paying attention to her mate, supporting his physical changes, reaching for more intimacy even as their sex drives eased. She screwed up her courage and asked him what was sexy, what made him feel loved, and the answers surprised her. It wasn't about her looks but about what she did for/to/with him. It was more about their emotional connection.

Her mother and grandmother have been wonderful role models for the ins and outs of aging. "People love being around them," she says. "They are fun and curious and interested in other people. They have an insatiable desire for new adventures and challenges, so they always have something interesting to talk about."

Although she has friends who get grumpy and depressed and whine about needing plastic surgery, she has little sympathy for these women. "If they don't like what they have become, why not do something about it and quit complaining?"

Jane has exercised all of her life and she is philo-sophical about the diminishing returns she now sees from her daily workouts. She has always eaten healthy foods and never really had to worry about her weight. "Since I began to go through menopause, I see the numbers go up on the scale and my waist thicken no matter how hard I try. I used to think that if older women would just work out and eat well, they wouldn't age. Now I see it's unavoidable."

Perfect love sometimes does not come until the first grandchild.

With her lifetime devotion to health and fitness, Jane was surprised to be diag-nosed with uterine fibroid tumors. She flatly rejected her doctor's assumption that she should have a hysterectomy. "Too many physicians' attitude toward post-menopausal women is 'You don't need this organ anymore anyway.'" Instead, she researched her situation and changed her diet to eliminate wheat and dairy foods, took herbs, and improved her stress management with meditation. "I stuck with it by picturing myself lying on the gurney in the operating room having a hyster-ectomy. When I went back to the doctor, he was amazed that the tumors had shrunk. Later, I learned that they typically shrink at menopause anyway. It's an estrogen thing."

Jane does not worry about the future and she is *really* looking forward to having grandchildren. She has wonderful role models. Her mother and 88-year-old grandmother make wonderful travel companions. They even did an all-women trek into the Grand Canyon last summer.

Jane is content. She is healthy and wants to stay that way. She does not mind being this age. "I can truthfully say that this is the happiest time of my life," she says. She sees her life as a major accomplishment and feels happy and serene. Like many of her peers, Jane has worked to educate herself about investments and has budgeted well. She and her husband changed financial advisors until they found one they feel comfortable with, who gives them the information they need to make good decisions for themselves. Now Jane feels financially secure and that she can grow old with grace and style.

Although she does not attend a church regularly, prayer has always been a central part of her life. As she gets older, she finds herself increasingly interested in spiritual affairs and has enjoyed taking part in a regular nondenominational discussion group. Jane is positive about her aging and embraces growing older. She contends her attitude defines her behavior, how she sees the world, and how the world sees her. "I spend less time worrying about what others think and more time finding other women who are positive and have good minds," she says. "Continual learning is key to successful aging. I stay up on what is good to read and stay current in world politics."

She used to paint, but stopped when her kids were little. Lately, she has picked up her paintbrushes, gone back to class, and is amazed at how fast it is all coming back to her. She felt so good about a recent watercolor still life that she donated it to a local charity auction — and *it sold*.

. . . .

JANE IS THE BEST PREPARED of our Fifties Women to enter her later years. She is the rare and fortunate woman who seems to have no reservations at all about growing older. She is in great shape due in large part to her active lifestyle. Because she has many great role models and has continued to learn throughout her middle years, she is eager to reinvent herself in each new stage of her life. She makes a good point that it's important to mentor our sons as well as our daughters. Boys need guidance to develop into the kind of sensitive, caring men that today's young women expect as partners.

Women like Jane have developed a deep trust with their husbands after many years together. They have learned to cope with their slower sexual responses by taking more time and experimenting. Secure in their relationships and enjoying their husband's desire and attention, they don't ask or care about what's normal because what they have is *great*. Jane says she feels good about herself when she has great sex or spends time creating art.

Living by the old adage, "use it or lose it," Fifties Women can enjoy everything: painting, workouts, career development, and, especially, a blossoming sex life. Even women who never resented the years of catering to a family's needs will happily seize this time to rediscover their independent, light-hearted, and quirky sides.

Women like Jane who take charge of their finances and investments actually make some of the best investors. Women are smart and savvy about which products work well and are loyal to their companies. For example, for years Jane's mother used Tide and now Jane does, too; she also has bought stock in the company and in others with that kind of name recognition and customer loyalty.

Women friends — including sisters — play an important role in maintaining mental health. It helps to learn other women's views and to have female role models to learn from. When a woman is happy with her age people often tell her how young and outgoing she is and that she is fun to be around. Who wouldn't want to spend time around people with those qualities? Jane seeks friends who are honest and trustworthy, possess a goodness of character and openness to others, and who have a good opinion of themselves. In general, women in their fifties believe that genuine people with good personalities, openness, and warmth make good friends.

WHAT DO FIFTIES WOMEN WANT?

As members of the Baby Boom generation reach their middle years, researchers say that many still hold onto the idea of being youthful past the age of 50 years, as if they were frozen in time. Even Baby Boomers age 50 and older say they consider themselves to be middle-aged. These numbers would suggest women see themselves living to be 100 years and older. And why not?

The fifties are a time of extremes for many women. Women who did not fear aging reported it was a positive rite of passage for them. But nearly half of Fifties Women say they are afraid of growing older and many of them are struggling. A lot of their fear is not for the present, but for their futures. In their fifties, a whopping 91 percent of women said they are confident of their ability to take care of themselves today. Fewer than 60 percent felt confident that they would still be able to care for themselves 20 years hence. This is disturbing because these women will only be in their seventies, a time that most healthy women are still vital and active.

Many women have worked to conceal their anxieties about their aging process because no one they know ever talks about it. This silence is unnecessary and destructive. They can benefit from honestly sharing their feelings and experiences about growing older.

WHAT TO EXPECT AFTER MENOPAUSE

- ❀ No more messing with sanitary protection
- ❀ No more fear of pregnancy
- ❀ No more avoiding white pants
- ❀ Time to adjust diet, exercise, and sleep patterns
- ❀ Vaginal tissues become thin, dry, and less elastic (vaginal atrophy)
- ❀ Reduced lubrication during sex
- ❀ More susceptibility to yeast infection
- ❀ Untreated, fragile tissue become inflamed, and tear and bleed during sex, making intercourse uncomfortable
- ❀ Insomnia
- ❀ Changes in shape and texture of facial skin (including wrinkles, dry skin, and changes in coloration)
- ❀ Weight gain due to a reduced metabolic rate
- ❀ Reduced hair production

Increasingly, Baby Boomer women are rejecting the superficial social values that say a woman must "Stay young and beautiful" to be loved. They feel their internal clocks tick-tocking and they are old enough to know the score: Ready or not, they are aging. Mother Time is making her mark and they want to do the most they can with the second half of their lives. They are acutely interested in being vital, sexual creatures and are not afraid to explore these areas.

FINDING AND KEEPING HEALTH

Fifties Women are now finding ways to accept that their bodies are no longer young; they have changed in ways that are simply impossible to ignore. The average onset of menopause, which officially occurs 13 months after the last menstrual period, is age 51, but some women do not reach that milestone until nearer 60.

What is Menopause?

Menopause is actually the thirteenth month without menstruation, so you are menopausal once you have not had a period for 12 months. The average age is between 50 and 52 years. Women may have stopped seeing a gynecologist after their childbearing years ended, but this is a good time to make an appointment for a checkup. Talk with a doctor you trust who can explain clearly how the changes you are experiencing may affect you.

Contrary to popular belief, menopause does not bring an increase in depression; the women most likely to get depressed are ones who already had trouble with depression earlier in life.

Women commonly report at least a temporary loss of sexual desire, perhaps partly because of embarrassment about their changing bodies; partly because of reduced estrogen levels; and for many women, the surfacing of long-buried relationship issues. Although most women continue to be sexually active late in life, around 20 percent of committed couples have a low-sex or no-sex union, defined as fewer than ten sexual encounters per year.

The denial of the forties has given way to the reality of serious health concerns. By the fifties, poor lifestyle habits like smoking and overweight are taking their toll and creating major health concerns. Gaining weight seems to be a big issue for many women as they enter this age group. The passage into menopause, which brings slowing metabolisms and loss of estrogen, creates inevitable body changes.

GET SCREENED EARLY AND OFTEN

Like it or not, risk increases as we get older. The best defense is basic prevention measures and a faithful screening program. Catch it early and there is a great chance of surviving into a healthy and vital old age. And although no one would ever want a serious disease, women who have come through the fire say that the experience changed their lives for the better and make aging itself look like a wonderful alternative.

Women often do not get the same level of care as men, at least partly because they do not demand it and because society traditionally undervalues women. They should not settle for second-class treatment, and they should stifle that little voice that says, "Oh, I don't want to bother anyone."

EMOTIONS OF FIFTIES WOMEN

- ❦ Acceptance of the change
- ❦ Rage if you've been repressing your anger for years
- ❦ Yearning for time for self
- ❦ Grieving the lost look of youth
- ❦ Frustration at physical changes
- ❦ Ambivalence and confusion in the face of strong emotions
- ❦ Confidence in own opinions and ideas
- ❦ Determination to make a difference
- ❦ Courage of her convictions
- ❦ Pleasure in sexual freedoms and expression

OVERCOMING HEALTH FEAR PARALYSIS

. . . .

When women feel powerless and over-whelmed, they may ignore signs and symptoms that may indicate a serious health issue. Here's what to do:

- ❀ Make your health examinations a top priority and get them regularly.

- ❀ Listen to your body and trust your gut. Women are extremely intuitive and know when things are not right.

- ❀ If you experience changes in your normal sleep habits, appetite, energy levels, and general feelings of well-being, see your doctor.

see sidebar next page

They should stick up for themselves. If they have any doubts that their doctor hasn't come up with a correct diagnosis or recommendation, they should get a second opinion. Doctors who suggest they are overreacting should be replaced. Good communication is the key to developing a team approach to maintaining health and achieving early diagnosis and treatment of any problems. It is OK to fire doctors who do not put their patients' wishes and concerns up front.

Fear is a persistent emotional response for many Fifties Women. Many women are afraid they will be unable to afford health insurance when they grow older, especially if they become unable to work. This fear often causes women to ignore their symptoms and delay seeking treatment. When treatment does not begin until a later disease stage, recovery is more difficult and less likely.

Women who are afraid of aging tend to have a greater number of physical concerns than those who are not fearful, although the types of health issues are quite similar. Fearful women do have significantly more abdominal complaints, but that's about the only difference in the pattern. High blood pressure, arthritis, fibromyalgia, diabetes, bone loss and degeneration, and back and hip pain continue to be common complaints for Fifties Women.

Women often reported more superficial problems such as aches and pains and losing energy and not feeling motivated. Women in general did not talk about their fear of breast cancer, heart disease, or other diseases that kill women every year. These variables suggest that women may often ignore their true health risks. Health professionals and family members should encourage women, especially in their fifties, to put a top priority on prevention and education about their health risks.

Fifties Women are seeing many of their friends and family members develop serious health issues while they themselves are seeing new problems turn up in health screenings. What is especially worrisome at this point is that Jane, Ruth, Betsey, and Sarah have all failed to mention the key health concerns that are killing women of all ages, largely because they may be more concerned about their families, friends, and careers than about taking care of their own healthcare needs.

The truth is, women often overestimate their good health and underestimate their risks. They are misinformed about their risks for specific age-related diseases such as heart disease and cancer. Even though half of all deaths are caused by heart disease, women's greatest fears were of getting breast cancer. This is not good, because women who don't get the right information about their risk for disease may make wrong decisions about their health and about their preparations for aging.

. . . .

I laugh, enjoy beauty, and love accomplishing a task!

. . . .

The good news is that public awareness campaigns have raised awareness in recent years about heart disease. Women have gotten the message that good health doesn't have to hurt! Many women have confronted their fears by becoming more proactive and devising strategies to stay healthy

OVERCOMING HEALTH FEAR PARALYSIS

. . . .

- ❧ Be your own best friend and advocate for your good health.

- ❧ By getting regular checkups, eating a healthy diet, exercising regularly (cardio and weight training), and managing stresses effectively, you are building a healthy foundation. If you do develop a health problem, your healthy habits will help you fight off the disease and recover your normal good health quickly. Be nice to yourself.

and active. The lucky women may be among those who will successfully celebrate their hundredth birthdays with their families.

Researchers have found that the women over 45 who were most unhappy wished they had made career changes that would have enabled them to better care for themselves as they grew older. Well, guess what: It's not too late! Every woman has the power to improve her situation.

Establishing an Exercise Program

- ▨ Set your goal and start taking baby steps.
- ▨ Pick a form of exercise you enjoy and can do easily and inexpensively.
- ▨ Write out the pros and cons and keep the list where you can see it.
- ▨ Be accountable: If possible get two friends to commit so at least one of them will be available.
- ▨ Keep a journal or log to record your progress.
- ▨ Reward yourself for achieving each baby step.
- ▨ Allow yourself to lag now and then. You don't have to be perfect.
- ▨ Get back on track after a time away.
- ▨ Consider hiring a personal trainer who will help you stay on track and keep you motivated.

CAN YOU RELATE?

Like women of every age, Fifties Women are concerned about relationships, both how to be in them and how to help the people they care about handle their personal problems. The old saying, "The hand that rocks the cradle rocks the world," shows how much women have traditionally been defined by their relationship to their children. As women enter their fifties, however, things really change. Most of their kids are off to the local junior college or university, or they're working or married; honestly, if they are still at home they should be *asked* to leave. Nearly half of all Baby Boomers have experienced divorce. Women who said they feared aging are concerned about their own sexuality, about what that means as a woman grows older, about their changing bodies, and also how men are doing with their changing bodies. Many women also deal for the first time with long-buried relationship issues.

I just keep learning and growing. I look forward to the time I get to do what I want. I want my own time.

Some relationships continue to be highly sexual; others cool. Not every couple is worried about this cooling, however. Some are relieved to at last take a breath and not worry about sex. Particularly as they get older, many women are more interested in having companionship with their spouses than sex, and they see their mature relationships as having more endurance and longevity.

Women who are concerned about their declining sexuality or physical discomfort can talk to their gynecologists and consider topical estrogens or other medical assists. In addition, good communication can help air old grievances and give both partners an opportunity to be heard. If both partners want it, there is no reason a couple should not be able to create a satisfying level of intimacy throughout their life together.

Fifties Women also want to clarify their relationships with girlfriends, co-workers, and other family members. What worked when they were 30 and 40 may no longer work in their fifties. When Fifties Women look at their relationships overall, companionship with friends, spouses, and family is a high priority. Many of them are shedding any relationships that don't have a lot of depth because they now understand what they need to be happy. They want to spend time with people who make them feel good and have enduring friendships that are healthy and fulfilling. They no longer want to put their own needs

FIFTIES WOMEN WANT OTHERS TO KNOW

❀ I am still a vibrant, sexual, interesting person with much to offer.

❀ I'm confused. How I look outside and how I feel inside no longer match.

❀ I want people in my life who are real and that I can trust.

❀ I get tired trying to please everyone. I want to stop worrying about their feelings and focus on my own.

❀ I am determined to have my words heard and respected.

❀ I feel like I am disappearing when I am disregarded and dismissed.

❀ I am concerned that people will think I'm getting too old to do my job and pass over me.

see sidebar next page

FIFTIES WOMEN WANT OTHERS TO KNOW

. . . .

❧ I sometimes want to run away from *all* my responsibilities and people who want things from me.

❧ I want to continue to dream and travel, have fun, and fall in love again.

on the back burner of life. These women are saying, "It is my turn at life," and "World get ready, here I come."

Women clearly understand they are different than men in so many ways, including the ways they handle stress. Throughout history women have been together…always working, but with lots of time trading over the back fence, or quilting, or cooking. Researchers suggest that women naturally tend and befriend. This tendency is highlighted in an anonymous Internet posting that circulates every year around Christmas: "If the Wise Men had been women they would have asked directions, arrived on time, helped deliver the baby, cleaned the stable, made a casserole, and brought practical gifts." Today women are in trouble because they are more isolated and have less opportunity to befriend each other. They are trying to compartmentalize their feelings (like men) rather than tending and befriending each other.

Women in their fifties can find comfort if they band together with other women as they head into a new era of their lives. Most women believe other women are doing better at aging than they are, when in reality, most women have doubts. In particular, those who worry about being wrinkled and old instead of cute and cuddly may take comfort from knowing others feel the same. Together, they have a good gripe session, then find a positive purpose for their maturing skills and abilities.

Face Up To It

. . . .

Women can help each other deal with feelings about their changing appearance by having an honest discussion. Get a copy of the video *Let's Face It* (www.letsfaceit.tv).

🦢 Watch the film with family or friends.

🦢 Wait to comment on the film until after watching the whole thing.

🦢 Start the discussion by telling each other one at a time about your experiences while watching. What did you react strongly to? What was familiar? What was startling? When you listen to others, notice your own judgments of what they say.

Choose among the following questions for further discussion:

🦢 What comes up about your face as a result of watching the film?

🦢 How do you see yourself in relation to the prevailing cultural values about maturing faces?

🦢 What messages were you given by family members?

🦢 What do you before you go out, and for whom?

🦢 How far are you willing to go to be attractive? Is cosmetic surgery an option?

🦢 What values do you wish to guide you as you evolve with your changing face?

Many Fifties Women said they could only guess how their mothers viewed aging issues. In earlier generations, most women simply did not talk about aging. They swallowed their frustration and their daughters had to guess what was on their mothers' minds. Other women said they did in fact have great role models, an auntie who wore purple and danced whenever possible. It helps us all to know how others meet new challenges.

FINANCIAL HABITS TO ESTABLISH

🌸 Depend on yourself.

🌸 Do it now instead of putting it off.

🌸 Blast your fears away with facts.

🌸 Select your goal and chart a direction.

🌸 Invest in your career.

🌸 Have a Plan B in place when your marriage ends through death or divorce (they all do).

🌸 Find and follow good professional advice.

From WIFE.org

WORKING FOR LOVE; LOVING TO WORK

Money clubs and investment clubs have helped many women learn about budgeting, investing, and retirement planning. Retirement (which I prefer to call healthy reinvention) is very much on the mind of women in this age group. Many worry about job security because of their age and wonder how they measure up to their co-workers. The lucky ones have developed new, marketable skills and have used their experience and knowledge to leverage themselves higher in the workplace. They are doing a great job caring for themselves but also know that a simple turn of events could bring them face-to-face with the responsibility of caring for aging parents or grandchildren.

. . . .

I think less about my appearance
and more about my abilities.

. . . .

SUCCEEDING AT THE AGING THING

Women feel successful when they feel energetic, vibrant, and youthful. All Fifties Women feel younger than they look, and they do well to accept the reality that their insides no longer match their outsides. One group of women made a video program about their changing faces. Some women have made up ceremonies that helped them grieve their lost youth and move on.

A psychologist and counselor may help if a woman is having an especially difficult time that she cannot resolve by talking with other women. Several women also commented on society in general needing to have more accepting attitudes toward older women and felt terms such as 'crone' or 'old lady' needed to go away. They felt they deserved a lot more respect and kindness and that their experience and knowledge seemed to be ignored, even though this was no doubt their greatest attribute.

Many Fifties Women have become completely comfortable with themselves and have stopped worrying about what others think of them. They reject the exaggerated modesty of their mothers and grandmothers; if someone catches a glimpse of their petticoats, so what? In fact, many of today's fashions require wearing your underwear on the outside. Fifties Women are determined to make their health a top priority and put their own health needs first.

They are comfortable in their skins and even as those skins change, they can make the leap to successful aging. They take their native planning ability and make aging a project that they are determined to manage successfully. At this age women have learned to value their native insight and instinctive abilities.

·····························

Be who you are today. Be who you are tomorrow. They need not be the same.

·····························

Many Fifties Women are also very good now at evaluating healthy relationships and know the value of good friends and healthy companions. Women say that success is based upon good planning; healthy attitudes and good friends; and staying healthy, being spiritual, and having strong values and hoping for the best.

Women in their fifties and older have spent much of their lives caring for others, and they are accustomed to ignoring their own needs. "Dr. Mom" needs to give herself permission to nurture herself for a change. This is not just a feel-good recommendation, either. Women in general seem to be in denial about their true risk of healthcare issues such as heart disease, lung cancer, diabetes, and other degenerative diseases.

Women in their fifties are also pretty realistic about themselves and know more or less how they want to live the rest of their lives. Many women have developed strategies that will help them live successfully throughout the aging process. Getting and staying healthy seems important to most women even if they do not address key concerns, and they want to have good companions and continue to maintain good psychological and spiritual habits.

Dr. Nancy's Kick-Butt Keys for Fifties Women

- Strengthen your relationships with friends, children, relatives, and associates.
- Speak the truth to yourself and others.
- Get proper medical care.
- Get serious about financial planning. It's not too late to start or improve.
- Stay active. Volunteer and give to others.
- Keep learning and growing.

- It's your life and your time. Stop making excuses and take every possible opportunity to do what *you* want.
- Grant yourself time to reflect on your life and your goals.
- Wish you looked better? Invest in self-care: take better care of your skin, exercise more, eat better, get more rest, or consider cosmetic surgery if you like.
- Seek out a good role model to teach resilience.

If a person thinks small and expects little, that is what she will get — each and every time. By reinventing herself as a big thinker and a real doer, the Fifties Woman is also challenging other women her age — or any age — to do the same.

Like Jane, so many women spend years taking care of others' needs and put their own needs on the back burner. Fifties Women are ready to say "what about me?" Women who do not ask will not receive, so it's time to gather their courage and cash in their sweat equity. Time to find their groove and make the dreams they have put away come true: paint, tap dance, travel, start that new business, find that new, satisfying relationship. They should not just sit back and wait any longer.

Today, Baby Boomers — Americans born between1946 and 1964 — are establishing many biological and sociological trends and challenging the very idea of aging itself. This group alone represents the largest single growth of the population in the history of the United States. As the sixties approach, those women are determined to create positive experiences for themselves. The oldest of the Baby Boomers are more than 60 years old and are helping to define both the job market and what their next stages of life will look like.

Visit www.womenspeak.com to learn more about the fifties. Express yourself and share ways you have learned, grown, and found your best life.

CHAPTER 6 *The* **60s**
Finally, Me First —
You Can Wait

I am having a wonderful time dating two men after my
divorce, but sometimes I still wonder just who I am.

VANESSA, 64

Although Sixties Women increasingly notice the effect their advancing years has on their bodies, most say they don't feel older until they glimpse themselves in the mirror. They startle and wonder momentarily, "Who is that person?" The image in the mirror doesn't match their mental self-image. They feel 30 or 40.

A woman who celebrates her sixty-first birthday today can expect to live at least another 23 years to become 84. Many will live much longer. Most women today believe they are not as old at 60 as their grandparents were, and with advancements in health care, nutrition, and opportunity, that is likely correct. Many women in this group reject society's negative view of the older woman. Interestingly, nearly half of people aged 65 to 69 still consider themselves to be middle-aged, as do many in their seventies. The Baby Boomers who are just entering their sixties certainly do not consider themselves old.

Many have evolved in their relationships and feel a balance and partnership with spouses. Others have opted for the single life. Still others have excelled in their careers. Most are now less concerned about what others think of them, and are more comfortable with dancing to their own music. Even though their mirrors remind them of each passing day, many are discovering better health than ever in their lives, greater inner peace, and a deeper connection with their spirituality.

Many of these women are not slowing down at all; instead, they are putting their careers in high gear and finding joy as they allow their passion and purpose to drive their choice of activities.

WHAT SIXTIES WOMEN WORRY ABOUT

By working on their mental health, they have learned to manage their baggage from life's disappointments. They feel a little dismayed at the continuing changes in their bodies, but mostly they focus on being glad they still feel young inside. It annoys them to find themselves treated differently, and many of them determinedly reject stereotypical age-based ideas about what they should wear or do. Overall, they are happy with their growing maturity and would not trade it for youth even if they could. Sixties Women see their knowledge and experience as premiums, their prizes for 60-plus years of living large.

Sixties Women feel successful when they keep a positive attitude and outlook on life. Living in the moment rather than worrying about past or future is a solid coping skill that helps them deal with tragedy or other life challenges. Sixties Women often refocus on their spiritual faith and find a renewed determination to follow their personal moral compass for being a good woman. Many of them discover a renewed purpose in working to make the world a better place.

Role models continue to be critically important, as do focusing on others and being able to assist and mentor. Sixties Women treasure friendships and relationships where they can give and receive love; indeed, their volunteer service forms the backbone of many social and community organizations.

Sixties Women are committed to staying fit and active with a lifestyle that allows them to pursue their interests and activities. They use their experience to sharpen their mental capability, including their ability to discern the ridiculous manipulation of advertising pressure about their aging appearance. Although women in their sixties still want to look good, they are more often able to reject the influence of advertising; they trust their intellect and life experience over the pressures of the market place. More and more Sixties Women now face real health challenges, both for themselves and with their aging parents at the same time that they enjoy being grandparents and becoming close friends with their adult children. Their increasing maturity gives many an abiding kindness, compassion, and sweetness.

Sixties Women resemble Fifties Women in that the vast majority of them are living full and satisfying lives. Even so, women in their sixties have the highest rate of health concerns of any age cohort, with two out of five saying health is their major concern as they get older. Money is a major concern for fewer than one in five Sixties Women, suggesting most either have their plans in place or are in denial. However, they do worry about being able to care for themselves and keep from being a burden on loved ones. This issue has a lot to do with retaining mental capacity, although just 10 percent named their psychological well-being as their major concern.

Although three-fourths of women in their sixties reported they did not fear aging, a solid quarter of them are afraid. A common thread of loss has started showing up in the fabric of many of their lives: loss of partners, friends, and family members. They regard their old parents with awe and some dread imagining their own turn at old age. Relationships continue to evolve, some for better, some for worse, and fewer than one in fourteen express any concern about being alone without a mate.

In this chapter, the composite profiles of Sally, June, Evelyn, and Mary demonstrate that for Sixties Women, life still offers infinite possibilities. They seek challenges and growth and, far from being ready to retire, many are working to expand their career opportunities. At times they are confused to still feel young while their birthday number grows and they wonder if they should act or be a certain way. Although each woman has her own distinct life pattern, all women share common experiences in this decade.

SALLY: "I FEEL WISE AND POWERFUL."

Sally, 66, divorced 30 years ago and never remarried. It hadn't occurred to Sally that her husband wouldn't keep his marriage vows. She didn't even care if he took a lover as long as he didn't rub her nose in it. They had made a commitment to each other, she thought. So it crushed her when he demanded a divorce. In fact, it so shook her faith in the institution that she has never remarried.

"Divorce is one of the best things that ever happened to women as long as we are able to earn a living on our own," she says. "Everything about my life has been better since my divorce, and I see no reason to tie myself legally to another man."

Now, she says, "I feel wise and powerful. I know who I am and like what I see, especially the inner me. My hair is definitely getting grayer and I tell people that those are threads of wisdom and that I am getting wiser every day. My biggest bodily concern is the way I am spreading out around my middle."

She is not afraid of the process of getting older, but she does fear being old. "I worked hard getting older and I'm going to enjoy every day of it! I expect to have at least twenty more active, healthy years. To me, old is when you are no longer able to do the things you want to do. It's a loss of energy and agility, horrible aging skin, and dementia. That's not me, so surely I'm not old!"

She worries when she feels limitations in her physical abilities and her energy level, and she gets angry that she can't seem to get things done like she used to. "I am more aware of 'Time, the Thief.' But as an artist, I think my work is far better now. Like most people, I didn't give much thought to aging when I was younger. Now that I see my 92-year-old father living a good and happy life, I hope I can do the same in my old age. I have to tell myself not to have a pity party.

Having seen so many changes in her sixty-some years, Sally remains an optimist. She believes that options for an aging population are going to increase. "I believe solutions we don't even know about will be developed. I can't believe 'they' will let us perish unassisted."

· ·

I concentrate on staying active mentally and physically, and hope that I will age gracefully.

· ·

Sally's greatest worry is being alone. For the past three years she has had a partner who is eight years younger than she and very trim. This makes her painfully aware that "my tummy bulges too much, my thighs are beginning to have that awful dimply look, and my legs have too many veins." She tells herself she needs to book an exercise class and "halt some of the damage," but somehow she never gets around to it. "Then I end up berating myself for letting my body go and know I should have done something about my tummy sooner but I got slack." She feels guilty and inadequate for not following through.

She worries that her younger partner will not find her desirable. She thinks a lot about sex, especially how to keep improving with age and its new physical limitations. She has worried about her changes in drive and function and has been willing to adjust expectations to get in line with reality. It has been a relief to her to learn her reduced desire is normal and does not have to spell the end of a satisfying sex life. She wants to stay in the game at least as much for her own pleasure as to please her younger partner. She likes her doctor well enough, but did seek another opinion about improving lubrication and the use of hormones for improving her sexual desire.

After her divorce, Sally realized she was dissatisfied with her job in day care. She completed an education degree and now works as a middle-school art teacher. She loves the students but finds dealing with administrators and the occasional unreasonable parent exhausting. Cutbacks in funding threaten to reduce her job next year to a part-time traveling position. "I worry much less about people not accepting what I do at work — and at home! It's more of a "so fire me!" attitude. I don't care. I have options and can always take early retirement." Despite her late start, she has a little pension built up, and she has been taking on a few private students in a home studio. This creates scheduling conflicts with her partner, who is around the house a lot.

Even so, she plans to enjoy herself taking part in groups with seniors, enjoying cerebral pursuits, and having time to meet others and go the beach. Sally craves new challenges and strives continually for lifelong learning. "In my twenties I had a group of older and younger women who loved and supported me, in my personal life and in the workplace. I loved working even though when I became single and moved to this town, all I could find was a three-quarter time job for $8,000 a year doing Mother's March for the March of Dimes (this after I had been earning $24,000 in a larger city). My father moved from Iowa to be with me; he is now 92 and waiting for a pacemaker. It's been a blessing to get to know him as an adult. I'm now the age my mother was when she died. I was angry that I got diabetes, but then decided that I must embrace my own body, which is a vehicle for doing great things for me. I used to hate my fat middle, but now I don't care. My favorite thing is people. Health is my major aging issue."

Sally's beloved female relatives have all had a terrible time with aging, which she finds a bit daunting. "Mother died at 30. I saw my favorite aunt living alone with Alzheimer's in deplorable conditions in her seventies. My other aunts and my maternal grandmother each had a hideous aging process and died in nursing homes with severe rheumatoid arthritis, strokes, ovarian cancer, Parkinson's, and heart attacks. Maybe that's why trying to make plans for the future makes me pretty uncomfortable.

"On the positive side, I think Erik Erikson's concept of 'acceptance of the fullness of the complete life cycle' has influenced me most powerfully." Happily, her inheritance from her father's side is much stronger. "My uncle lived and died with dignity and natural acceptance that I admire! And Grandma was straight and proud at 77, which was great. She had suffered much pain for her loved ones but still loved life. It broke my heart when she declined rapidly after 80 and then died."

For Sally, improving her self-image requires her to feel and look smart and energetic. "All of us were beautiful when we had the bloom of youth, but then you start having things happen to you: wrinkles, bags under eyes. My hair is not only silvery and beautiful…it's thin! I could be overwhelmed, but I prefer to face it and accept it."

Feeling good about herself means getting up in the morning, ready to face whatever the day will bring. "I love telling the truth, nurturing my friends and my students, and shopping! I like it when someone compliments an outfit that I am wearing or a new hairstyle, and I love to luxuriate in the royal treatment of a spa. But there is just no satisfaction that compares to completing an art project and knowing it's a good piece," she says.

Sally worries about dementia taking her mind. "Of course I am concerned about my looks as I get older," says Sally, "But what is most important is my mental stability. I worry about my ability to control my own destiny." Because of watching her aging relatives fail, Sally has educated herself about wellness and nutrition, and strives to avoid doctors and prescription medicines at all costs. "I feel like our healthcare system actually promotes more sickness. Prescription drugs so often do not heal the body but only treat symptoms and many have serious side effects. My body is my most valuable asset and I will not turn over responsibility to someone else. I want guidance on how to live a healthier lifestyle."

Despite her pursuit of health, end-of-life issues increasingly cross her mind. "I used to wonder if my partner, who is much younger than I, would be willing to assist in taking care of me if my health got to where I would need help," says Sally. "I decided I do not want to be a financial burden on him or anyone, so when the time comes, I have decided to go to a nursing facility and I am paying the premiums on long-term care insurance."

· ·

SALLY FACES MANY CRUCIAL ISSUES as a Sixties Woman. Like all her peers, she has to come to terms with the personal loss of her physical youth and beauty. She looks at her family history of multiple health concerns and wonders if she will follow the same pattern. In the background of all her other choices, she has lingering questions about the stability of her committed relationship with her younger partner.

Unlike some of her peers, women like Sally understand and calmly face their choices. Because they do not want to burden others, they are ready to deal with several issues. The advancing years make them wonder about their ability to care for themselves later in life, and they often wish they had prepared better and earlier to provide for their financial security. By obtaining her teaching credentials and moving into a professional career, Sally implemented a plan of action for her financial and health needs. When a woman has watched poor health affect aging female family members, she needs to try to keep her focus on family members who provide a good example of successful aging. Family history does not irrevocably determine one's fate, but it can provide warnings and focus attention on useful preventive measures. Sally's fears are real; certainly no one is in a hurry to experience the declines of old age. However, she does not need to obsess about potential future losses.

Sally's strengths lie in the fact she is well connected to others and she can reach out and get help from friends. Friends can help a woman find answers to her concerns, including taking a more active role in managing health with good nutrition and exercise, locating a financial advisor, and continuing to plan for eventual long term care needs. A Sixties Woman's greatest asset by far is the ability to recognize the need to get her act together now, while she still has time to plan for her future. By increasing her education and qualifications, Sally has moved into a teaching position in public school that came with health benefits and a secure pension, both of which will provide her with a more stable financial situation later, when she is no longer able to work. Women who recognize that their security depends on these actions are miles ahead of those who remain in denial about growing older and who avoid thinking about their futures. As each step in their plans develop, they find they sleep better and have a greater sense of calm. Sally is smart and other women could learn much from her example.

JUNE: "NO ONE ELSE SEEMS TO STRUGGLE WITH AGING."

June is afraid of getting older *and* of dying. Now 61, she has spent her life being scared of lots of things. Widowed in her early fifties, she was shocked at how quickly death changed her life. She had never balanced a checkbook or handled any of the family's business affairs, so she had a crash course in taking responsibility for herself. Now, she works as a church secretary, where she deals with aging and death on a regular basis. She dreads the changes in her body and frets over every new wrinkle and spot.

"I am worried about leaving my loved ones," June says. "I think about aging but I keep very busy to avoid worrying." She is involved in many activities through her large church, but when she stops her frenzied activity, her concerns quickly surface. Her family history is not good and every aunt or uncle has died of Alzheimer's or other dementia. Her closest aunt developed Alzheimer's at 52 and died of it at age 62. June has feared this her whole life. She doesn't want to be like them and has even had a MRI scan to check her brain status.

"My biggest problem with aging is memory loss. I know I'm not quite as alert or quick-thinking as I used to be, especially when I'm multi-tasking. I'm OK if it's in my BlackBerry, but I'm in trouble when I forget to enter it. I'm concerned about being forgetful. Is it normal, or am I being like Mom? My doctor says I should cut back, that I just have too much going on and I am on overload. He suggested I try that for a year and see if I still have trouble, but I don't think I can wait a year to find out I have a real problem. When I think about my age and compare myself with my family I really get scared. Women in my family do not live long by today's standards.

"I'm almost as old as my aunt when she died, so I'm better off than she was. But I worry that I will lose my physical and mental abilities. I think about getting older most of the time, when I talk with my friends about aging and most often when I am alone.

"My mother is absolutely negative and rejects the natural aging process," June says. "She was widowed at age 62 and remarried less than a year later. My father had been four years younger than she, and she was supersensitive about her age and filled with shame that she was older." At church, June's mother announced that she would stop coming before she would go off with the older group. "She gets her hair fixed twice a week, and is more focused on clothes and makeup than ever before in her life. Now, she is an irritated, angry, resentful caretaker of her older second husband who has Parkinson's disease.

"My mom complains constantly and has become bitter and nasty," June continues. "She plays the victim role and does not enjoy her life. The innumerable hours she has spent in church seem to have produced absolutely no spirituality and no peace. She is consumed with fears and anxieties about everything — storms, earthquakes, bugs, snakes, accidents, planes, news, murder. She wants to be in control of everything, which of course is not possible!" The thought of the loss of her loved ones — and there have been quite a few — can depress her terribly, and she tries to avoid thinking about it.

....

*Aging is part of life. Consider the alternative:
I would rather "get older" than die young!*

....

June says she found out what it is like to feel invisible after becoming a widow. "It's not just about looks, though," she said. "This is a 'couples' world and a woman alone is discounted and often ignored." It enraged her to feel that no one wanted what she had to offer. Even at work, she feels she is relegated to petty, minor roles when she could offer so much more.

Her loving and caring relationship with her daughter is her most important personal connection. "My daughter and I spend a lot of time together and that really makes me feel good about myself," says June. As important as this relationship is, June's appearance is still a dominant part of who she is. In her youth she liked the positive attention her looks drew from men and women, including her mother. "Now I think I look like an aged person," she says. "I don't look as good in my clothes as I used to, and I just do not seem to have the willpower to diet." She worries about her weight, hair loss, loss of her youthful bloom, wrinkles, and sagging muscles. June says, "I would like to be able to grow old gracefully... but it is so hard to do." Her self-image is also very important to her and she wants to "look put together for an older woman." Reacting to her mother's example, she wants to have a nice personality and not become a grouchy old lady.

June remarried three years ago, like her mom, to an older man. She has experienced some problems adjusting. Deeply reserved, she says, "I refuse to talk about sex with anyone; that would be a betrayal of my husband." In truth, June thinks sex is for younger men and women, and that a Sixties Woman who has any sex life at all should be happy. She wouldn't dream of asking her husband to take an erectile dysfunction medication. She shyly confides that she really does not have a strong desire for sex and sees her aging body as another sign to just let it go and not worry about it any longer. Since her breast cancer surgery, June really does not like to look at herself. "What man would want to look at me either?" she asks.

Her breast cancer affected her self-image, but her daughter has been impressed that her mom took it so well. June was used to working on her looks, so putting the prosthesis in her bra each morning is little different to her than getting her hair colored to hide the thinning and the gray. She enjoys getting a manicure and pedicure, uses good skin care and natural cosmetic products to help her face look pretty and decrease her wrinkles, and dresses in attractive clothes that accent her best features. When she does these things, she feels she looks inviting and exciting to be around.

For the most part, June battles her fears alone and tries to keep on keeping on. "No one else seems to be struggling with their age, and I'm afraid my friends will think I'm just being silly. They tell me that surviving breast cancer should be enough of a reason to be glad each day I'm alive." Yet for June, it's not enough. She says, "I wake up in the morning going through my mental checklist of what I have and don't have and wonder about my future. It makes me so tired I want to go back to sleep and not think about anything."

June would love to have someone she trusts who would listen to her concerns and help her plan a healthy life style, but she does not feel her doctor listens to her. "It's as if he lost interest in me when I passed childbearing age. Sometimes I feel ignored and dismissed." June really wants to stay independent and her health fears make her feel frustrated and vulnerable.

"I am concerned that the medical profession is becoming more dollar conscious instead of concerned about my physical care," she says. "I don't have the faith in the physicians of today that I did in my younger years. I wonder if Medicare will be there for me and if I will be able to pay for prescriptions in the future. And I don't really understand the drug benefit." "I'm afraid the politicians will really mess up Medicare and Social Security," she says. "As it is, I'll be in trouble if a big unexpected expense comes up, such as a new furnace."

June worries in a general way about her ability to care for herself in the future. She often thinks with dread about developing a handicap, especially with her history of arthritis, and it's a prospect that angers and depresses her. "Will I have the energy and the physical and mental ability to live a healthy and productive life?" she wonders. "I especially don't want to deteriorate to become a burden to my daughter. Sometimes it feels like all downhill from here."

Her financial future looks uncertain. She had a little money set aside for retirement but her first husband died without insurance and her salary does not quite cover her expenses, so her small savings are still being eaten up. "I need to keep working and yet I see a day that I will not be able to do my job. This is a big concern and I really should talk with a financial advisor to start my retirement planning."

. . . .

ALTHOUGH JUNE FEELS ALONE, SHE definitely is not the only Sixties Woman trying to figure out this "growing older" process. An important first step for any woman is to improve her health and exercise program and successfully meet other life challenges. This can help get rid of fears of aging.

A woman who lets her fears block her from living a life full of passion and purpose is in danger of sinking into a downward spiral. If she settles for a job that does not challenge her, she may allow her life to shrink steadily as she grows older. Allowing fear to rule will keep her shortcomings as the focus instead of her opportunities and strengths. Women who are too hard on themselves may become immobilized from a constant stream of negative self-talk and worry about what others will think.

June has experienced many losses. Her husband died when she was in her fifties, and she now perceives she has lost her youthfulness. She feels alone. Although she has remarried, she does not appear to feel supported and sustained by that relationship. June also lacks a positive role model. She feels burdened by her mother's misery and fears she will end up the same way.

The realities of life may lead women who bear heavy burdens to feel discouraged and hopeless at times. By worrying continually and dwelling on their troubles, they leave themselves vulnerable to depression and an anxiety disorder. Physical health also may become compromised if they do not find emotional relief. In this situation women must find new resources to help with a spouse's failing health if they are to have any quality of life at all. The situation will only become more critical over time and they need to face their fears head on. Like many women her age, June lost herself a little at a time through the years until she came to fear change. But she's sick of that. Now June is ready to take risks and wants to feel that she can fly free of fears once more.

June would really like to have a life in which she is able to show others her talents. To do this a woman needs to build back her self-confidence so she can reject the negative views of society about being older or looking like an aging woman. When women get their power back they can stop dying on the vine and instead find their own rules for living. A strong confident Sixties Woman can tell everyone, "Get out of my way because here I come."

Fearful women like June also would benefit from a mental health intervention with someone they trust. Working with a professional counselor or psychologist could help June understand how her thoughts are affecting her emotions and her general view of the world. Cognitive behavioral therapy can help her to identify and deal with negative thoughts and irrational thinking, see things more clearly, and help her develop a plan to feel better about her life.

They also need to make plans for the future to ensure they can care for themselves and an ill spouse during the time he has left. Being in charge of all of their day-to-day needs, including health care and finances, is a lot of responsibility, and it helps to have a support group and resources, for today and for the long term. Finding ways to get away and make time for herself as her husband becomes more dependent will be important to June's mental and physical health.

It's wonderful that June has so many strengths to help herself out of her ambivalence about getting older. Women tell us that when they make the effort to look and dress well they often feel better about themselves. June's high level of personal energy is a real asset; she likes people and people like her in return when she makes the effort to get out of her woe-is-me routine. Having an outgoing personality is another asset because it enables a woman to connect well with others.

Women like June also are fortunate to have the assets of faith and a large church community. Strengthening their belief in a higher power provides a sense of peace and hope for the future. During tough times many people have a hard time finding strength but June has a golden parachute. She finds healing and sustenance in her daily meditation and prayers and this give her some ease from her fears and her worries.

Women who have not found any successful female role models to emulate may feel "out on a limb" and may lack coping strategies to help with aging fears. Despite her own fears, June's cognitive learning and spiritual development have put her in a much better place than her mom occupies. Although June fears aging, she at least would like to be able to accept it as a natural progression, much more so than her mother.

June also is aware that her daughter is watching and learning from her example and she wants to be a positive role model. Many women say they feel invisible at times and especially as a single woman after a divorce. Many women describe this feeling beginning as early as their forties, and by their sixties, they are learning ways to counteract it. Speaking up and having something to say are great ways to become visible; so is joking lightly with people to get them to take notice. It bothers any woman to feel left out and ignored when they have so much to offer.

A life coach can help a woman who is struggling to find the job she wants and to fulfill the potential of her God-given talents. Coaching can provide common-sense information that could help change a fearful, worrisome life into a life full of passion and promise. June also knows she needs to start planning her future. She often worries about not having anything to fall back on in case of an emergency and hates the idea of relying on the kindness of people at her church. Many women find the idea of asking for help so intensely foreign that they instead suffer silently, paralyzed by their unmet needs. Clearly, any Sixties Woman would have done better to begin her retirement planning 30 years before, but this is a common problem with many women who simply never got around to it.

June is not having much fun these days and spends many hours a day worrying instead of taking action and responsibility for her future. Women stuck in this pattern need to contact one of the many great organizations that help teach women in transition how to manage their own lives. June is ready to get started taking care of herself, and she finally believes that she deserves it and is worth it.

EVELYN: "I DON'T THINK OF MY AGE UNTIL I SEE MYSELF IN A MIRROR."

"I have a large group of friends ranging in age from 22 to 82 years," says Evelyn, 64. "So naturally, I have started to lose the ones who are older than I am. That's why I am trying to cultivate new friends who are a bit younger than I am. It helps to keep me active, laughing, and not as concerned about aging."

She does notice that younger women today seem to think more about themselves than she did at that age, and notes it's probably good that they are able to be more selfish. "I was one of the few women in business when I started, and we dressed for success and had to try to be like men to compete. Women today expect more than we did.

"I don't think of myself as an 'age.' A Chinese actor once said he would forget that he was Chinese until he passed a mirror. That's how I am—I don't think about my age until I catch a glimpse of myself. I didn't focus on my youth when young and I don't focus on my age now. I just look on it as a marketing obstacle because some people have age issues. But people don't focus on my age because I have too much energy. In the same way, when I was young I didn't want them to think about how young I was because that excluded me."

Evelyn began her career as a secretary, moved into middle management, then started a realty firm with her then-new husband. Now, as a veteran realtor, Evelyn feels strong and confident in her job and most years earns a good income. With her husband's support, she is cutting back to part-time work in their family realty business, partly because she has noticed a decrease in her energy. It takes more effort now to stay energetic and motivated. "There are so many agents now who are 'hungry' and willing to work long hours to get the contracts signed." Evelyn is no longer willing to work 24/7 and do anything to make a sale. These days, she follows up on referrals from current clients but leaves the pursuit of new business to the younger, more aggressive agents.

As she grows older, Evelyn is pleased to have less stress in her life, partly because she worries much less about what others think. She relishes finally being able to put herself at the top of her priority list. She was always "the one with the big voice" and just loves to sing at weddings and special events. Her goal today is to develop a second career as a gospel singer. She regards this as a stimulating, interesting business that can keep her engaged until she retires in 5 or 10 years.

Evelyn and her husband have been married for 38 years, and they enjoy a mutual affection and tolerance. Their long-term, successful relationship has deepened and broadened over time. "I think about aging when I long for more sex in my relationship and realize there's less and less time ahead for that enjoyment." Evelyn is adapting to these changes in her relationship in the same way she accepts the changes in her career. "Sex just seems less important to me than it used to and our spiritual bond, mutual respect, and loyalty seem even more important. We have become good friends in the best of ways, with admiration thrown in for good luck. That's not a bad way to live with a man, is it?"

Through the years their sexual connection has been an abiding pleasure and healing bond between them, and she feels fortunate they have been able to adjust to their physical changes with good humor, arriving at a place of even deeper intimacy. The trust they have developed over the years has enabled them to cope with their slower responses and they take their time and enjoy experimenting. Sex is good but no longer the driving force of their youth.

Their four children are grown with families of their own and her two sons live near by. These relationships with her children keep Evelyn feeling young. "I look forward to the fun times, loving times, calm, peace ... the serenity of knowing I have four beautiful children in the world who are all as loving and aware as I am, and they are on the journey of life with faith and hope." "My greatest concern is to maintain good health and see my grandchildren through college," says Evelyn. "I want them to be just as happy as I am, especially when they reach the age of freedom from all the cares they have now. I loved raising my family. I learned a great deal from so doing. But, I am happy to have at least a few carefree days now. I earned every one!"

She enjoys mentoring her daughters-in-law, both of whom appreciate her respectful treatment and light touch in their relationships. This brings all of their family together for both major events and everyday get-togethers. Sadly, both Evelyn's and her husband's aging parents have health concerns that require lots of attention. This takes time away from the many things they wish to enjoy, such as travel and spending free time with their children and grandchildren.

As a member of the sandwich generation, Evelyn does a lot of patient juggling. She and her husband continually modify their plan of action to find the time and the energy to keep their lives rational. Evelyn's mother, now 91, was a teacher when that was her only career option. "She is my role model," Evelyn says. "She always did everything she could do and didn't give up any freedoms until absolutely necessary. She made the best of every situation, never looked back, and kept moving forward."

Last year her mom developed serious health problems, including dementia, and Evelyn moved her mom into their home. Providing for her 24-hour care has made Evelyn and her husband confront all the issues of planning for what might happen to them in their own turn.

In this, Evelyn has a positive role model in her mother, and she is grateful her mom saved and planned for her eventual need for long-term care. Although her mom was a nurturer and caregiver her whole life, she was able to foresee a time when she herself would need help. She did not allow herself to feel defeated when she could no longer care for others or even herself.

Evelyn has been a pioneer for women and since she began her career, she felt it was important for women to excel in the workplace and be involved in decision making. She sees women as powerful and having the skills to bring about change. "I have been in business my whole life and I remember the days when there were no women in the Chamber of Commerce or in Rotary. I saw this as a waste of women's gifts and abilities, so I got together with other women to create a businesswomen's network. Singing is my fourth career and I have been excited and energized by each of them."

Evelyn has several real estate clients in their eighties and nineties who make good role models. "I have watched some women age really gracefully by staying active." Like many other women, however, she quickly runs out of acquaintances and resorts to celebrities. "I really admire Nancy Reagan. In spite of her long and tough journey, she has been an amazing role model for women. Also Katherine Hepburn, Tina Turner, Georgia O'Keeffe — any woman who takes deep breaths of life and inhales it all."

Evelyn admires women who keep their eyes lifted to a higher plane, and she is placing top priority on her own spiritual health. As she grows older, her faith and her regular prayer life have stepped up a few notches, although she still does not regularly attend church services. "I tell myself that with God, I can do anything, and that there is no rush in doing things," Evelyn says. "This is my time to do things in an unhurried way. After raising four children and rushing to meet deadlines at work, this is my luxury time. I tell myself: 'Time will take care of everything.'"

Evelyn seeks out the company of younger friends to help her feel young. She loves to be "with happy people having a good time and not sitting around talking about things I have no control over." Evelyn's list of things that make her feel happy is a long one. "Enjoying the smile of grandkids, great-grandkids and family, waking up in the morning without pain, incident or accidents." She loves waking up early praising the Lord and meeting people who are full of joy, peace, smiles, and integrity. Her power grows when she takes the time to pray. "I grow by praying with my prayer partners on the phone, continuing to learn and use my mind, and being involved with other people in ways that are giving and spiritual." All these things make Evelyn feel her life is well lived.

. . . .

Aging is not important. Living each day as it comes is all that is important.

. . . .

"I have vowed not to talk about the pain of getting older. No one wants to hear about your aching legs because theirs are aching, too!" She also is realistic, having watched so many others fail and drain their spouse's resources. "If I became incapacitated to an extent that I must drain family strength and finances," she says, "I'm ready to travel on to see what comes next after this life."

This is part of her preparation for what is to come after her death. "In the past, my faith and prayers have helped me when life, people, and the world have let me down," she says.

. . . .

SIXTIES WOMEN LIKE EVELYN WORKED hard to get out of the typing pool and find jobs that paid a living wage. They wanted it all, and fought against society's limitations and worked together with other women to expand their opportunities. They juggled their careers and kids and the house; many, like Evelyn, are now looking forward to being less busy and driven.

Evelyn is a great example of a woman who has had a good role model for successful aging. Having a positive role model helps women find their personal power early and learn to use it to challenge themselves and serve as great role models for their children, family, and friends. For women like Evelyn the keys to happiness are associating with positive and uplifting people, places, and things. They expect not only to be successful but to be happy and joyful about the outcomes. By continually challenging themselves to grow and evolve from one career to the next, they gain confidence, happiness, life success, and satisfaction in the connections with those they love. Evelyn admires self-made women who did not allow society to dictate how women should act, and be seen (as beautiful and well-dressed) and not heard (keep your views to yourself and better yet, do not have any).

Evelyn has done many things to empower herself and other women to join and grow in business. This step alone ensures that these women will be able to care for themselves whether they wish to marry or stay single. Evelyn is ahead of this learning curve and is helping other women to do the same. Women should not wait to take charge of their financial responsibilities.

For most women, the majority of a lifetime's healthcare costs accrue during their last year of life. Evelyn has always looked to her own mother for answers and now wisely learns by watching her mom's challenges with losing independence and failing health. It is clear to her that just as her own mother needs assistance, Evelyn one day also may need help.

That day is still a long way off, however. Although Evelyn is willing to endure what aging brings, she refuses to cling to life if the cost becomes too high. Women are fortunate when they have good communication and problem-solving skills in their relationships. For example, Evelyn and her husband feel sustained by their shared life and trust. They have talked honestly about their wishes and made living wills to help guide family members if either should become incapacitated. When women see the importance of taking matters into their own hands they plan carefully for their futures so they can avoid placing any burden on their children as they grow older.

Eager to start her fourth career in her sixties, Evelyn loves a challenge and thrives on change, which many other women and men find difficult as they grow older. Evelyn is better prepared than many Sixties Women to face life's challenges in a fluid and flexible fashion and she is ready to re-invent herself once more. By directly facing the issues of age women are better able to handle direct competition with younger, more energetic and determined women and men. They need to find their place and use their passion and purpose to energize their careers.

The keys for Evelyn's success are that she is comfortable with change or newness *and she expects to be successful.* She may find she can derive all the satisfaction she needs from her own version of a singing career without beating herself up that she can't become a Hollywood star. Women like Evelyn have learned an important life lesson that some women never learn: they have patience, they believe time is on their side, and they are willing to work and wait for their "good" to arrive. Meanwhile they filled their lives with people and projects that sustain them.

MARY: "NO ONE CAN MAKE ME DO ANYTHING I DON'T WANT TO DO."

Mary was the youngest of her four siblings. Now 68, she has never married. Instead, she has instead focused on her career and taken an active role in helping her aging parents.

"I'm too independent to put up with any man," she says. "For that matter, several of my women friends have wanted to share a house, but I can't see living with them, either." She helped nurse her father until his death 10 years ago and admires her mother's survival attitude. Mary worked 40 years as a middle manager for a federal agency. She did equally well supervising men and women, and felt that she had reasonably equal opportunity to advance, despite the preponderance of men in the highest ranks. "I think women are stronger than men," she says. "That's one reason they are so hard on us in so many cultures; men are threatened by our strength."

When I continue to learn and grow and laugh I almost always look forward to tomorrow.

Her government job gave her a solid pension and benefits, but she was starting to feel old around her younger co-workers and began to dread going to work. So eight years ago she retired to start her own online furniture accessories business. The business has done well, thanks in large part to her wonderfully reliable older women employees, and Mary is now semi-retired.

Mary is an optimist and works to maintain a positive attitude. "I realize that I can still participate in the activities I like, but I may need to adjust them for my age and health status." Like most women, she has some conflicting thoughts about getting older. "The aging process is not scary but the possible deterioration of my mobility is," she says. Her age has affected her ability to exercise and participate in sports and often she pushes so hard her body aches. "I think of getting older when my body isn't able to do something my mind can still embrace." Still, she pushes to maintain strength and fitness both for her own sake and so she can continue to be strong and active for others.

Mary's grandmother lived to be 98 and played basketball with her teenaged great-nephews on her ninetieth birthday. "The many lumps that life dished out never seemed to take away the laugh in her everyday countenance," Mary recalls. Her mother also has helped her to view aging in a more positive fashion. "My mother is cruising along at 82 with only one boyfriend now! She is a great role model for health and she continues to work out four or five times a week and she is very careful about her diet."

As a single person, Mary is always on the lookout for good examples to help with her aging process, both in life and in her reading. This is vitally important, she thinks. "I look for role models in magazines and books for reinforcement." Mary has adopted her mother's pattern of participating actively in lots of different groups, including church, cards, and travel, so she devotes little time to feeling lonely, tense, or down. She has never spent a moment worrying about finding a perfect "soul mate."

Her feelings about growing older parallel her mother's in many ways. "I do not spend a lot of time worrying about it, and she did not either," Mary says. "It's going to happen, so just be glad you're still here. My mother would have said: 'if you must worry, find something worthwhile to worry about and then do something about it.'"

Women who regard aging as a blast tend to see that, like growing up, it has its drawbacks, but not enough to ruin the fun. "I fill each day," says Mary, "and if tomorrow never comes, I have lived and laughed, and above all, I have loved away my life.

"Until this year I don't think my mother knew she had gotten old," says Mary. "She has been a big influence on me to stay active and never say 'can't.' Things just sometimes take her longer now. She went back to college when I was at university, got her degree when she was a grandmother, and when she retired she became principal of a religious school affiliated with her synagogue. She has always kept her focus on living.

"When women talk about feeling invisible, they're usually worried about being invisible to men," Mary says. "I don't care. And I look good, so it's not about being a dog. It is more important to me, however, that others realize that I am open to new ideas and am intelligent. I strive for acceptance, graciousness, understanding of others, interaction with others, and to continue life-long friendships."

Mary feels successful in her own aging process, and although she pooh-poohs appearance, she is pleased to look 10 years younger than her age. The best way to cultivate a good self-image, she says, is "by having character and being kind to others." She likes to spend time with her nieces and nephews and family and is enjoying her opportunities to travel, have leisure time, read, and explore.

....

I don't think of myself as getting older but as reaching maturity.
I am experiencing wisdom more than age.

....

"Worry ages you, so I live in the now," she says. "That is, I laugh at yesterday, and have no concerns about tomorrow. Today is mine, and I want only one thing ... to share my joy and love with other people." Going beyond herself helps keep her young, she thinks.

The list of things that help Mary feel successful and satisfied starts with being able to travel and do things, but then comes back to relationships. "I like to meet a challenge either at work or home that results from an ability to communicate with others. I have found that I always receive the assistance I need and usually accomplish my goal. I feel good when I can listen to the problems of my friends, and help them either mentally or physically."

Mary feels grateful for her general good health, especially when she thinks of her friend Jill, who has lupus, a chronic disease. Managing that has become a full-time job, and helping Jill has made Mary think a bit more about growing older. It has renewed her determination to remain as fit and strong as possible and to try to look realistically at risks she might have been ignoring. For example, she says, "A lack of muscle tone would mean I was in a danger zone for injury, and I want to avoid anything that might lead to my not being self-sufficient."

Mary occasionally jokes about getting older and having senior moments, but she takes this in stride. "When I can't remember a word in a crossword puzzle, I just go on to another word and when I go back a couple minutes later, I remember the word I had forgotten. I can still complete a computer jigsaw puzzle in the same or less time than younger people. It makes me realize that I can still excel in another way. I can keep up with my family, and interact with my great-nieces and -nephews! I am not getting old, I am getting better."

Her lifetime habit of positive thinking leaves Mary cheerful and upbeat. "I don't talk with anybody about my concerns. Talking about age and insecurities is a nuisance and distraction from things I'm interested in, and I don't expect to feel differently when things start getting worse. I don't ever focus on my weaknesses. I watch the various signs that my body is getting older, and I know them, but I see no reason to talk about them."

When asked what she looks forward to about getting older, Mary says: "I am there! I looked forward to being independent. To doing things when and if I wanted to! One great thing about getting to my age is there isn't any client who could make me do anything I don't want to do!"

Although many Sixties Women say they feel powerless in their sixties, women like Mary get fired up. "Occasionally I curse in private, and then I'll communicate with government groups and elected officials to try to effect change. I'm more politically active now than ever," she says. She takes personal responsibility for her county's politics now and works tirelessly in her local issues and elections. It gives her hope, helps her make connections, and makes her feel informed about the issues.

"It is onward to the next chapter of my life. I am willing to admit that I am entering the autumn of my life, but it's my favorite season, and I shall stave off winter!"

When she is not busy caring for family members, Mary thoroughly enjoys the benefits of being semi-retired. "I work just three- or four-day weeks now, so I can often sleep later, cook and eat when I please, and, at least part of the time, my attention can now center on me."

. . . .

MARY HAS LITTLE TIME FOR herself, but she has always accepted this as her role in life: to be kind to others. Mary is often all things to all people, and not having a spouse or children leaves her time and energy for her work and caring for others. She has a dream to have more time for herself; however, she worries that other people will think her selfish and lazy if she kicks back a bit. This is a common worry for Sixties Women who have driven hard all their lives to achieve many career and personal goals.

Women like Mary need to heed that inner voice to free up more time for themselves at this exciting stage of life. Sixties Women who can reduce their work schedule even slightly can make progress towards that goal. Women who have asked for little support from other family members should tap their families to assist with their parents' needs. This will give them respite and allow them more time for themselves. In addition they should investigate other types of assistance to help with this process. Even when a woman has successfully carved out personal space, her primary concerns include maintaining independence and meeting her own long-term healthcare needs.

Mary has many strengths and offers a fine example of successful aging. She enjoys her freedoms and credits her health and good situation to a life well lived. When women understand aging is a process they cannot out-run, they can make friends with it. This keeps them from dwelling on their losses or becoming depressed by all the implications of a changing body. Instead, they focus on their strength, on being in charge of themselves and being flexible. By accepting the role of caregiver for a parent who is also a good friend, a woman can remain involved and feel good about offering her services for the good of all.

Work-wise, women like Mary are called 'traditionalists,' because they prefer to stay with one or two employers for their entire career. They draw much satisfaction from a job well done, and they are very loyal. Mary is a doer and making the world a better place is high on her list of priorities. By remaining determined not to let her age prevent her from doing what she wants, a woman can keep a firm hold on her personal power, continue to express her own views, and refuse to become invisible.

As women rise in successful businesses they can delegate more and more of responsibilities and replace them with things she wants to do. Many women like Mary are finally giving themselves permission to take personal time to do the things they have put off or delayed because of care giving or job responsibilities.

Mary is lucky she has two excellent primary role models in her mother and her grandmother, which accounts for her positive attitude and absence of fear about aging. Women who calmly see aging as inevitable can go on with their lives. Many women are successful when they take control of their lives and see aging as a normal part of living rather than a disease that has to be cured. Women who keep a positive outlook are more likely to experience positive aging. Women who have had good role models as well as good mentors at work or in the community find aging to be a reward rich with experience and opportunities. Mary can be both role model and mentor for younger women and her nieces and nephews will benefit from having such a "cool" aunt.

Mary will no doubt continue to model herself after her own mother and grandmother's examples of successful aging, including coping with emerging health issues. In particular, her mother demonstrated that finding something worthwhile to worry about and doing something about it — in other words finding your passion and purpose — was a great way to stop worrying about things she could not change.

Sixties Women are successful with aging when they stay connected and continue to challenge themselves with new and interesting people. By maintaining a strong network of friends a Sixties Woman can advance her chosen causes, and remain caring and involved in others' lives without compromising her independence. They are especially able to balance their lives when they understand they are in the driver's seat making choices for themselves rather than being forced to conform.

Women like Mary also are successful in life because they are good communicators and know the power of bringing people to the table. Good communication skills and the ability to inspire teamwork are valuable strengths both on the job and in a woman's personal life. By bringing together others who do not like the word "No," women can accomplish much with their ultimate multi-tasking skills. Mary's enduring support system is her strong network of women friends, which is by far her most valuable tool as she continues to get older.

Mary lives a life that will ensure her independence and well-being. Women who realize their health is everything are ahead of the game. When they start early to take good care of themselves, and then continue to exercise, take vitamins and herbal supplements, meditate, and stay involved in the world by volunteering and being useful, they are likely to have good health into old age. Mary keeps up-to-date on new research and products and will do what it takes to stay on top of her health.

WHAT DO SIXTIES WOMEN WANT?

Sixties Women have a better than 50-50 chance of living another 20 or more years. They have a lot of living left to do and are just hitting their stride. They are wise, knowledgeable, savvy, smart and — if they choose to be — just as sexy as ever.

Sixties Women particularly are asking for things that should be a given for every woman: respect, consideration, appreciation, and the right to feel good about all their life experiences no matter what time has done to their bodies, or their minds, or their energy levels. Sixties Women are rejecting stereotypical thinking about older women and insist on re-defining themselves. Like their mothers before them, they are surprised and often amazed that being 60 feels like 50 or 40. As one mentioned with surprise, "I did not realize that my insides would not age along with my outsides." The image in the mirror looks out of sync with their youthful thinking and dreaming of things to come.

Sixties Women want it all and why shouldn't they? For an average 85-year lifespan, typical for a woman now in her sixties, the middle third of life ends around age 56, which would indicate the sixties are in the last third of life. But it doesn't feel that way to most women. Twenty-nine percent of women said "old" comes some time between the ages of 60 and 69. Although a few thought "old" happens even earlier, a majority of women view their increasing age numbers not as a negative but as proof of a valuable life filled with experience and knowledge to be shared. The older a woman gets, the later she pushes the "old" benchmark.

Many Sixties Women still consider themselves middle-aged, and will continue to do so well into their seventies. They plan to live well into their nineties … and beyond. One-fourth of Sixties Women say they are afraid of getting older and 40 percent said health was their major aging concern.

DOING AS SHE PLEASES

Sixties Women know themselves, and they have found so many ways to satisfy themselves and counteract life's discontents. Women are finding their voices as they grow older and they are finding they have saved up a lot to say about what they really think. Women in their sixties do like their newfound voice of reason and that voice now roars their true thoughts. Although each of our Sixties Women has a different personal style, more and more they shed their fear of "what will they think if I …?" and instead ask, "Who cares what I do? I have a right to express myself and no one is going to stop me."

Women who have a history of being decision makers, who are comfortable with and welcome change will age much more successfully than women who have spent their lives conforming to what they think society wants them to be. June is an example of a woman who believes that as she grows older she must settle for what is handed to her. She feels little ability to impact her life.

My own grandmother had warned me about society's judgments. When I would complain that someone disapproved of my actions (I was not a quiet one) she would reply; "You must have shown your petticoat." I got the message loud and clear that women who do not conform, who allow the "slip" of their individuality to show, often find themselves targeted with disapproval and exclusion.

···································

I look forward to doing what I want,
when I want.

···································

LOOKING FORWARD TO REFIREMENT

Sixties Women who still work enter a period of major change early in this decade. While close to half of women aged 60 to 64 are still employed, that percentage drops to just one in ten after age 65. The oldest of the Baby Boomers are Sixties Women now and are helping to define both the job market and what their next stages of life will look like. Although more women use their increasing lifespan to work longer years than ever before, retirement becomes a holy grail for many Sixties Women. They daydream about a long list of benefits: being wise, being looked up to as a role model, making a difference for younger people and their families, continuing to learn and do some things they did not have time for previously, and sharing their joy of living with family.

Yet for every woman who looks forward to settling back into a leisurely retirement, another plans to "refire" her life with new interests and excitement. Women are re-defining themselves and taking time for themselves, and often making our world better at the same time. A significant challenge a Sixties Women may face in retirement is redefining her identity: "Who am I if I no longer am working?" That's why I prefer the terms *reinventing or refiring* to *retiring*. Sally reinvented her career from daycare into teaching art, and she found new excitement about her post-work phase of life too. In contrast, men frequently continue to identify themselves in terms of their job, even after they leave it, which creates problems for them.

When I attended a five-day symposium on mid-life issues including how to find one's passion and re-invent oneself after reaching mid-life, I noticed that the majority of participants were in their fifties and sixties and spoke openly of their mid-life status. Because they still feel young and strong, these women reject the idea of "retirement" and replace it with the term "re-invention." Instead of retiring, they want to "refire" their lives with inspiration, finding their purpose and passion and making it their new career. Women are finding and putting excitement back in their lives and doing things they never thought possible. They are traveling to distant places, developing extensive networks of women who are doing amazing things to make the world a better place for women and their families. Women who have spent years working to earn are now taking their cash and putting it to work both for themselves and for the world. Finding their passion and purpose enables them to reach ever-greater levels of productivity and value.

Women are wise investors, and many have planned and budgeted carefully so they can get along on a reduced income after leaving regular employment. Sixties Women who started early will continue to make sound investment decisions throughout their lives. That said, nearly two women in five who are aged 65 and older are kept out of poverty solely by Social Security. More

HOW TO REINVENT, REFIRE AND INSPIRE

- ❀ Think of the great example you will provide for everyone around you.

- ❀ Find out what makes you feel good and what energizes you.

- ❀ Release that creative part of yourself: paint, write, dance, create a new business.

- ❀ Give time and talents to others to help them grow: become a Big Sister, mentor a young woman, coach someone at work, volunteer for a social-profit organization.

- ❀ Find your spirit guide. Meditate to explore within; hear your breath; find your soul and your higher power.

- ❀ Travel to learn and grow; come back and use it to make a difference.

- ❀ Connect and reconnect with others.

SIXTIES FINANCES: MAKING UP FOR LOST TIME

· ·

- ❧ Eliminate debt, especially expensive credit card balances.

- ❧ Scale down your lifestyle; get used to living on less and save any raises.

- ❧ Maximize withholding into retirement plans.

- ❧ Increase your income with a better job or second job. It is never too late to learn a new trade or skill or go back to school and begin a new career.

- ❧ Postpone retirement. Integrate your purpose and passion into your work and hang in there.

- ❧ Invest in growth stocks (with professional guidance).

see sidebar next page

than one in ten are poor *despite* their Social Security benefit. Women at 65 are likely to live at least 19 more years, three years longer than men. Planning for the future is no laughing matter and Sixties Women have more than a good chance of living at least another 20 years.

This is one of the clearest messages younger women can take away from these stories: they need to shrug off their denial and start planning and saving. Because most women will outlive their partners by several years, women need to learn about costs and availability for their eventual long-term care when they can no longer live independently. By talking with a good financial planner, Sixties Women can learn about their options and gain some reassurance and comfort for their futures.

Only a third of women over age 65 are married. Many women who depended on a man to make the things that go bump in the night go away discover that in the end they have to take care of themselves. It's a surprising truth that all marriages end, either through divorce or the death of one of the partners. Many women Evelyn's age did not handle their own finances until their man was gone and they were forced to take responsibility for themselves.

This trend may be fading in younger women, and Evelyn's children have an opportunity to learn from their parents. Women's futures will be more secure, as will that of their families, when they routinely learn to handle their own financial affairs, either alone or with a spouse.

Many women transition into a part-time home-based consulting business to ease into full retirement. Evelyn's friend Beverly did that, and when her husband retired a few years later, she faced a big adjustment. "He forgets that I keep a rigid eight-to-noon schedule," she says, "and he's driving me crazy. I know there's going to have to be a change — I feel it in my different attitude. At age 69, I'm not interested in building my business as I was at 45 and 50. Maybe 10 years ago I'd turn down seven out of ten prospective clients, now I turn down four out of five. I think about the things I have to do to close down my business, but then I think of my clients who are dependent on me. I haven't dealt with it yet; I'm just playing with it in my mind. When we think beyond five or six years, we've talked about going to live in Greece."

WHO IS HERE FOR ME?

The role models of our youth and later years exert a powerful influence, whether for good or ill. Women of every age face choices when it comes to dealing with these formative influences. They can follow in their elders' footsteps and emulate their example. They can react to what they saw while they were growing up and do the opposite. Or they can pick and choose, charting their own unique path through life. The more alternatives a woman has been exposed to, the more likely she is to be able to map out a life that is uniquely satisfying to her.

My mother worked hard to open doors for me. She helped me get better jobs, and opened new career paths. She made sure I knew my body belonged to *me* and that I could choose whether or not to reproduce. But Sixties Women also see we have much to do in the fight to end poor pay rates, gain entry into top managerial positions, and end age discrimination for older women.

SIXTIES FINANCES: MAKING UP FOR LOST TIME

. . . .

❀ Invest regularly in retirement savings. If you invest $5 a day at a 9 percent return (maybe someday we'll get returns like that again):

~ In 20 years you'll have $100,000

~ In 35 years you'll have $440,000

~ From age 22 until retirement at 65, you'll have a cool million dollars.

~ If it's too late for this option to work for you, teach your daughters and granddaughters; they'll thank you!

From WIFE.org.

Evelyn's children have had a great role model for good relationships and they all share similar values. Research has shown us time and time again that women who have had positive female role models excel and are successful in the key areas of finance, relationships, health, and aging successfully, that is, without fear and negative consequences. Sally focuses on the good example of her father's healthy side of the family, while remembering the need to provide for a possible decline like her mother's family experienced. June's only role models are the negative examples of her mother's fears and aunts' health problems.

Many women in our study indicated their fears of aging mimicked that of their mothers, aunts, and other female family members. They often felt confused or fearful because of their exposure to their mother's negative, fearful views of aging while they were growing up. Women with fearful role models may have a rougher time, but they can overcome what they have been taught.

Many Sixties Women had mothers who didn't talk about their feelings. They often have no direct knowledge of how their mothers felt about getting older and must make assumptions based on observation. Women need positive role models to understand the elements and tasks necessary for successful aging. Women who struggle tend to know little about aging or have watched a mother or family members struggle with, deny, or even laugh away this important developmental stage.

Bridging the gap between generations is a challenge for most women. Sixties Women are beginning to "get it" and know that younger women do not, in fact, "have it made." Young women say they want mentors yet don't know how to reach out to the older women whom they admire yet who intimidate them. Older women who feel ignored and discounted by younger people can work on their communication skills. Unless the young women are complete brats, taking a genuine interest in them and asking questions will help to draw them out. Their inexperience leaves them feeling uncomfortable. It's not realistic to expect them to excel in gracious conversation, plus, they probably can't imagine what someone in her sixties might do with her time. If all this sounds like too much work, it's perfectly acceptable for Sixties Women to just relax and be themselves while the young women chat about their own interests.

Emotions of Sixties Women

- Feeling sad at losing her younger self
- Wondering how much time is left to fulfill dreams
- Worrying about relationship with partner
- Excitedly making time for herself
- Wondering about her health and self care
- Refiguring her finances and wondering how long she will have to work
- Wanting to use her passion and purpose to reenter the world
- Want to make a difference and leave a mark
- Seeking greater spiritual peace
- Planning her coming years to have time to do more for herself
- Feeling confident about herself and her decisions
- Having wisdom and ability to let others be themselves
- Eagerness to continue growing and having new adventures.
- Determination to continue as a sexual being who deserves intimacy

Women need to understand that they can directly influence their daughters, friends, and all women with whom they come in contact. By talking and sharing with other women, they can gain understanding and clarity about the ways society's negative views of aging affect women's self-esteem and self-image.

LOOKING GOOD MATTERS

It's a rare woman — of any age — who cares nothing for her looks. Although appearance has slipped far down in the priorities of most Sixties Women (in fact it has fallen below everything but their concerns for family), a few women in this age group still mention their looks, wrinkles, gray hair, and loss of energy as their major aging concerns.

While many Sixties Women said they care less about what others think of them, there's a strong sense of wanting to preserve personal dignity. They'll say, "I generally make sure I don't wear things that make me look like I'm trying too hard, or trying to look like something I'm not." They don't want to appear foolish.

The vast majority of women deal reasonably comfortably with the changes age brings to their appearance. They may not like it, and many avoid mirrors as much as possible, but they accept it. However, a tiny percentage of Sixties

SIXTIES WOMEN WANT OTHERS TO KNOW

. . . .

- 🌸 I want time for me — you need to wait.
- 🌸 I want to have lots of passion and purpose in my life.
- 🌸 I want to relax instead of and worrying about what you think and what you want.
- 🌸 I dream of things I have not done yet; I do not want to have any regrets.
- 🌸 I am afraid my body will let me down and I will not be able to care for myself.
- 🌸 I am afraid I will not have enough money to live if I do not work for the rest of my life.
- 🌸 I get tired and want to slow down and just be by myself.

see sidebar next page

Women — just two out of one hundred — selected "losing their youthful appearance" as their major aging concern. This is a terrible burden our youth-obsessed society has placed on these women because this is a losing game. Nothing can eliminate the signs of passing years on a woman's skin, body, and mind, although conscientious self-care, sun protection, exercise and a positive attitude can help her stay healthy and strong.

Other women are using science and complementary medical procedures to look their very best as the years begin to show. Many say, "I do not want to look younger but I do want to look as good as I can and have my insides match my outside." Women have choices and many are OK with lines from laughter or the extra pounds and have learned that true beauty is much more than a pretty, unlined face that has nothing to say. All must find new ways to feel good about themselves despite their changing appearance.

As Baby Boomers enter their sixties, they are on their way to setting yet another record. Almost half of all married Baby Boomers have already undergone a marital split. This means Boomers are virtually certain to become the first generation for which a majority experienced a divorce.

Sally's comment that divorce is one of the best things to happen to women reflects society's changing views of women's opportunities. I have worked with many women who had never written a check for themselves until their husbands asked for a divorce. Sally was told she had to sign up for some kind of class — even at the local technical school — in order for the courts to order her ex-husband to pay maintenance. Long story short, she took a medical transcription course and now has people working for her. She likes herself, she has slimmed down, her kids are now grown, and she's excited about her new opportunities. A lot of people find it invigorating to discover they can take care of themselves despite their apprehensions.

One last note about soul mates: this fantasy concept has caused a lot of unnecessary pain and angst. Every woman in every relationship is going to face trade-offs, no matter how wonderful her man and no matter how ecstatic she may appear. In real life, we take the good with the bad. If the good is good enough, we may be able to overlook the bad almost entirely. But don't kid yourself that the bad is not there. Women should be honest with themselves about their relationships and the short list of what they need, keeping the core list clearly in mind and not worrying about a "perfect" soul mate.

One-fifth of single-person households in 2000 were women ages 65 and older, and older women are much more likely to live alone than younger women or men of any age. This will probably continue to rise as women realize they can do this themselves. In fact, many more women today do not marry at all. Lawyers tell us that increasingly they choose to be in committed couples, including same-sex relationships, and they use prenuptial agreements and relationship contracts to spell out their arrangements.

Sixties Women have learned that living alone does not have to equate to loneliness. Women learn from each other and gravitate into groups of women to listen as well as express what they think.

SIXTIES WOMEN WANT OTHERS TO KNOW

* ❀ I am still sexy and even if I have a few sags, I can still be romantic and fun and exciting.
* ❀ I want to be respected and appreciated for who I am and what I do.
* ❀ I want to be heard and never feel dismissed.

A wise woman will bow out, however, if a group just sits around and complains, because she knows she needs to spend time with positive people to build a positive life.

Women's creativity is endless, as is the list of reasons they get together. Women who want to make a difference can look around, notice what their communities need, and do something about it. Join a board of directors to meet other women like yourself who are involved and passionate about making a difference. Financial concerns unite women of all ages, who instinctively understand that financial stability will give them power and control over their own futures. Women's athletic associations bring women of all ages out to have fun and network for present and future business endeavors.

Travel is an excellent way to learn, grow, and build self-confidence and self-esteem. Banks and hospitals have recognized the fact that women like to travel together and organize many opportunities for local, regional, and even world-wide travel. Politics and religion are crucial to any healthy society. Gather with other women who share your beliefs and work for your common goals.

There's no limit, so start today. Share the organizing chores, share rides, take turns hosting, and don't worry about the dust.

Women Get It Together

If you don't see a good reason below to gather together with other women, make up your own.

- Money Clubs or investing groups.
- Girlfriend weekend getaways: to the city, country, spa
- Girls' night out — or in
- Mentor women in your profession or the wider community
- Women's athletic clubs: bike, hike, swim, golf, work out, or play.
- Food-oriented groups: ethnic dinners, wine or coffee clubs, monthly lunch or dinner meetings.
- Political groups that educate women on the issues and help get out the vote
- Hobby groups: Books, gardening, sewing, knitting, crafting, scrapbooking
- Faith group: Bible study, or study of world religions
- Memory keepers: write memoirs, make books

✍ Cards or board games

✍ Business support groups: meet at breakfast, lunch, or dinner

With aging come the much-publicized losses: youthful beauty and energy ebb, friends and family members pass away, physical agility shares the stage with aches and pains. Many women also lose their identity and purpose when their care-giving roles or meaningful employment disappears.

Sixties women work on their coping strategies with greater or lesser success. Most women say they are healthy and express no particular concerns. Their concerns center less on money than on a possible erosion of their ability to be self-sufficient. End-of-life issues, which they had mostly disregarded before, frequently rise to the top, often because they are helping their aging parents prepare for death.

Sixties Women like Sally have acknowledged their possible future needs and are making plans to pay for nursing care or long-term care. Many stay in jobs they don't particularly like in order to keep their health insurance. Others — often ones like June who have little financial leeway in their budgets — are in denial and postpone beginning their planning process until well into their sixties. Feeling powerless causes them to ignore the future and not think about it.

Sixties Women worry about how they will pay for the ever-increasing costs of healthcare. Although Sixties Women for the most part still feel healthy and strong, they need to work harder at it. Regular checkups and screenings are critically important, including mammograms and Pap tests (no matter what their age or whether or not they have completed menopause and are no longer ovulating).

Although all four of our Sixties Women have either planned for their financial needs or spend time worrying, Mary's friend Jill, who has lupus, has let it go. "I don't really worry about my finances," says Jill. "If I don't have enough sense to live on what I have, I am liable to have some 'skinny' months! I can't spend what I don't have and in looking around I have seen that if I get to where I can't take care of myself, someone will."

Women are in the major league when it comes to multi-tasking, and Sixties Women worry a lot about declining energy and motivation and forgetting small details. Some forgetfulness is a normal part of growing older, but the brain needs to be exercised just like muscles do. Women can develop strategies to help them

KEEPING YOUR MIND SHARP

. . . .

- Exercise and keep physically fit.
- Eat a diet rich in antioxidant fruits and vegetables and Omega 3 fatty acids.
- Get enough rest.
- Read, learn, and grow.
- Do routine things in a new and different way: Shower with your eyes shut; drive a new route home.
- Surround yourself with interesting people.
- Travel to experience new and exciting things.
- Do things that challenge you: learn a language, try a new job or skill.
- Volunteer and interact with others.
- Keep up with current events.
- Manage your stress level.

with memory and planning and execution of everyday tasks, including making lists and reminders.

Keeping physically healthy is the key to the best possible performance and keeping disease at bay. Mental health also is important and goes hand in hand with overall health of the woman.

Women are four times more likely than a man to be diagnosed with a form of depression and/or anxiety. (The criteria used to define depression emphasize female-gendered behaviors such as crying and feeling sad; men do not admit to such behaviors but many more commit suicide than women, indicating they probably experience undiagnosed depression.) Women have much of their identity locked into their roles as caregivers and when they are not able to accomplish these tasks, or this task is no longer needed, many women will face an identity crisis. Those who have suffered clinical depression earlier in life may find that it returns. Sixties Women usually find their hormone-related emotional changes have leveled off somewhat, although physical changes and declining energy levels can leave a woman feeling sleepless and blue. Women who swallow feelings of loss and hopelessness and guilt and anger and direct them inward also are at risk for poor self-image.

Betty Freidan was a pioneer in examining women's health and aging issues. She noted that aging was being treated as a disease, and an incurable one at that. She found that the medical community often discounts physical complaints and aches and pains as just inevitable symptoms of aging without offering support or any recommendations for prevention or treatment. It is ironic that as their healthcare needs increase, women may find that attention from physicians decreases. Although many aging women are happy with their doctors, others find that their healthcare providers are pretty unavailable. This may encourage them to discount their symptoms and not seek medical attention. This may be one of the primary reasons women, especially older women, may ignore or deny important health concerns. This is a problem because it places them at unnecessary additional risk from conditions such as cardiovascular disease, stroke, cancer, and the ever-increasing type II diabetes. Smart Sixties Women feel empowered to "fire" a doctor who does not adequately address their concerns and shop for another one.

NORMAL AGE-RELATED MEMORY LOSS OR DEMENTIA?

Normal age-related memory loss	Dementia
Forgetting names you remember later	Memory gaps that impair daily living
Forgetfulness stays about the same	Forgetfulness gets worse
Forgetting words	Forgetting how to do things you've done many times before
Forgetting the name of a blender	Forgetting how to use a blender
Telling someone a story again	Repeating phrases or stories in the same conversation
Did I pay that bill?	Difficulty handling choices or money
Slower to learn new things	Can't learn new things
What did I come into this room for?	Doing things that require steps, like a recipe
Forgetting which day you did something.	Losing track of what happens each day

Other reasons women ignore their health risks may be that they are too busy taking care of other people, or that they truly don't realize what their risks are. Ignoring risks is not the same things as holding a positive thought. Faith, for example, works wonders but cannot replace regular medical care and self-care. Evelyn's religious faith is a rock upon which she leans. June finds support in her faith community. People who believe in a higher power deal better with injury, illness, and life's hard knocks than those who do not have faith. They not only believe in themselves but have the faith and knowledge that they will be cared for

HEALTH PRIORITIES FOR SIXTIES WOMEN

....

❦ Get a check-up.

❦ Make sure you have a healthcare provider who will listen to you.

❦ Exercise to improve your energy levels, self-esteem, and self-image.

❦ Connect or re-connect with others, rekindle with old or make new friends. Get involved in your community.

❦ Get out of your rut. Do something surprising every day with people who like new adventures.

❦ Travel to expand your horizons. Grow and never stop learning.

❦ Do something for someone else; make this a better place to live.

see sidebar next page

and that what will come is for the good of all. Having faith keeps them from fretting and worrying.

As Boomer women continue to reinvent their lives, they need to reach out to educate themselves and others about their true health risks. One woman suggested, "We need to develop an area of education information — perhaps groups through senior centers and bring humor into all of it. Help people look at the aging process through better channels, including men who think that they need a young woman to feel like a man again."

IT CAN'T BE ME TURNING 70!

Developmentally, Sixties Women have faced many of life's major changes, and they are now spending more time on the whole issue of aging. Children have grown, marriages have ended in divorce or death, or have changed as both partners reach their maturity. Health has become a major concern, and finances, physical ability, and energy are their primary concerns for the future.

Sixties Women feel most successful about aging when they view it in a positive fashion and see it as a passage and a natural process. Women who feel less successful felt shame and surprise at feeling invisible in a society they feel no longer prizes them as much as when they were young. Many Sixties Women are becoming more realistic about aging and no longer are allowing the media and the market to sucker them into buying products that promise to "make them look or feel 10 years younger."

Women also are turning to spiritual comforts and finding ways to build good self-images. Though many of these women reported not having good aging role models, many said they are actively seeking resources and examples that would help them to better understand and deal with aging.

Most women know that they do, in fact, need to be proactive about their aging. They believed that by staying healthy with good diets, exercise programs, and daily use of vitamins, and by being involved in their own health care and financial planning they would be more successful at growing older. As they look across the fence at the seventies, many women who have not faced it before begin to realize that they need to make plans for caring for themselves.

Dr. Nancy's Kick-Butt Keys for Sixties Women

- Live in the present but remember the good times.
- Relish the benefits of age, including senior discounts. You've earned them!
- Be a good friend and mentor others.
- Take time for sharing and caring.
- Stay sweet. Don't go sour!
- Exercise for flexibility, endurance, and strength training.
- Value yourself enough to eat right and stay healthy.
- Keep your working groove going for as long as you can to feel young and vital.
- Incorporate your passion and purpose into your work if possible.
- Associate with friends and family who love and appreciate you.
- Plan your financial future and work your plan.
- Each day, look your best (hair, skin, clothing) and you will feel your best

HEALTH PRIORITIES FOR SIXTIES WOMEN

- Find your personal power and make your life about your purpose and your passion.
- Be happy and satisfied and have an attitude of gratitude.
- Surround yourself with beauty and people who make you feel good.
- Get rid of clutter; clear out anything you do not need or use, including toxic people.
- Connect with your higher power and meditate, find peace, center yourself, and let the small stuff go.

Sixties Women can build on their past experiences to propel them forward along their own paths. They can choose: "Will I be a victim or a victor as I move into my seventies?"

Visit www.womenspeak.com to learn more about the sixties. Express yourself and share ways you have learned, grown, and found your best life.

CHAPTER 7　　*The* **70s**
Welcoming Wisdom and
Loving Life

My grandkids are amazed I am going to China this year.
They wanna be just like me when (if) I grow up.

JOYCE, 71

Most Seventies Women have adapted well to the aging process although they still don't like the toll taken by the passage of time. Women who have been vital contributors their whole lives express annoyance at the lack of respect they are beginning to feel. In groups, they find themselves sidelined as if they were uninteresting, and they may feel their expertise is not appreciated. In contrast, however, their value and ability to contribute within their own families rise as their retirement (which we prefer to call the refiring or reinspiring stage) brings increased availability for caring for their grandchildren. Some Seventies Women are now thinking about their passion and purpose and finding ways to give back to world during their next life stage.

Despite the common stereotypes of aging, most Seventies Women still feel healthy and strong, considering. Their minds are sharp and they are interested in their lives and their futures. A woman who celebrates her seventy-first birthday today can expect to live at least another 16 years to become 86. Many will live much longer. Many meet the suggestion of retirement with strong emotions and they may feel insulted to think they are no longer needed.

Some Seventies Women express surprise. They didn't expect to live this long; they still feel young inside; or they thought their health would be better. As a lifetime of ignoring chronic health conditions begins to take its toll, the old saying runs through their minds: "If I had known I would live this long I'd have taken better care of myself!" Seventies Women may suddenly decide to exercise and eat right, and they can derive immediate benefits.

In addition, many Seventies Women feel a bit confused. Just how are women in their seventies supposed to act, especially when they feel much younger on the inside. They say, "If I did not look in the mirror every day, I would never feel older; I feel young and vital and excited about the possibilities and adventures waiting for me."

Although most Seventies Women would by now admit, albeit grudgingly, that they are getting old, one-third of Americans in their eighth decade still consider themselves to be middle-aged. They still feel young and still see themselves as younger than their mental image of 70. They have many more years of living to do and may take up a new career, hobby, or interest. Many women say, "At last I do not have to be accountable to anyone else."

WHAT SEVENTIES WOMEN WORRY ABOUT

Nearly all Seventies Women said their declining energy levels frustrate and annoy them. Women in their seventies are definitely eyeball to eyeball with the realities of growing older.

Whether they voice it or not, Seventies Women are thinking — if not worrying — about their ability to take care of themselves in the future. They are increasingly reluctant to make predictions about how they'll be doing even five years into the future. More than three-fourths of Seventies Women now accept growing older with a measure of calm, but nearly one in four is afraid of getting older. Nearly 17 percent say their greatest aging concern was not being a burden to others. About equal numbers (14 percent) of Seventies Women mention being alone without a mate or having health problems as their major aging concern. More than nine percent of women aged 70 and older mention finances as their major aging problem. And the same percentage of Seventies Women (nine percent) select "psychological well-being" as their major aging concern. A mere three percent still consider their appearance to be their largest aging problem.

Seventies Women feel most successful with aging when they find ways to stay usefully involved in the lives of others. Having saved and planned carefully for their old age, they are now able to make ends meet without anxiety, even if it means living on a very tight budget. When they make it a priority to keep their minds and bodies healthy, they derive the benefits of feeling well and being able to do most of the things they find meaningful. The most successful Seventies Women continue to pursue their own interests, learning and growing, and they follow their curiosity into exploring new things. By maintaining a positive attitude, even if some of them face chronic pain and struggles, Seventies Women are determined to enjoy this important decade. Other women in their seventies are doing even more: they are going forward as if they knew without a doubt that they will live to celebrate that one-hundredth birthday.

Maintaining a sense of independence is crucial for most Seventies Women, even if they are living with family members or in a retirement facility. Although they may need various types of assistance from time to time, they want and need to continue to make their own decisions regardless of their living situation. Maintaining self-control and self-confidence is key for Seventies Women who want to feel competent and successful in their later years.

In this chapter we meet Dorothy, Virginia, Barbara, and Shirley. Their composite profiles reveal the energy, excitement, and zest that women continue to feel as they grow older. These women meet their challenges with strength and resolve balanced by the wisdom gained through years of varied experiences. They find their mentors in younger women as well as women in their eighties, nineties, and one hundreds and it annoys them terribly to be discounted as merely "old." They know how to choose their battles and appreciate the beauty and joy of a single hour. With luck they are comfortably reaping the rewards of a lifetime of good planning and decision making.

DOROTHY: "I JUST WANT A LITTLE RESPECT."

Dorothy, 77, has leased a small house ever since her divorce 20 years ago. Ten years ago she retired from her clinic job as a psychiatric social worker and now volunteers more than 40 hours each week as director of community services in a program for indigents. She actually wears many hats in the organization and loves working. "I just want a little respect; I don't need rewards or public recognition but I love it when someone says, 'Thank you for what you do.'"

Dorothy is living an enviable seventies life: she has good health and the energy to care for herself and the people she loves. "Although I love what I do,

I also really want to travel. I have considered the Peace Corps or doing mission work for my church. I want one more adventure.

"I'm not at all worried about aging," Dorothy says. "I have less apprehension than when I was 40 or 50 and I can accept the process. But I do have concerns about being incapacitated at any age such that my care would become a hardship for my children, that I might be a burden and that I will not be ready to accept the pain or disability. I'll try to cope with whatever comes along, and my first priority is to remain independent."

She looked into assisted living and just didn't like it. Her son has asked her to come live in an apartment adjoining their house, an offer she is considering. "The reality is, in 10 years I'll be 87, and I can't gauge my psychological and emotional functioning that far into the future."

Dorothy's mother lived a long, healthy life and still enjoyed gardening at age 90. "I loved my mother and grandmother," she says. "They both lived up into years but we never talked about aging. Mom never talked about her feelings much, even when she was dying of cancer at age 95."

Although Dorothy plans to emulate mom's longevity and good health, she doesn't accept her mom's attitudes about aging. "It's a different time and a different social milieu. My mother was a typical housewife of the Thirties and Forties in the Midwest. She was the only girl in a large family and was the family slave, so she spoiled me!"

Like many women of her time, Dorothy's mother found her options to be quite limited. She understood as she entered womanhood that she was expected to leave her parents' home, marry, and live happily ever after. If it wasn't so happy, she just kept her mouth shut. She did not talk about her real experience of getting older and shared none of her feelings and concerns with her daughter.

Dorothy's experience as a working single mother in an Eastern city has been quite different. In her urban life, Dorothy has looked outside her family to find many strong, smart women for role models, including two women from her church. "They were immigrants from Guyana who died in their nineties," Dorothy recalls. "One was the matriarch of a large family; the other was active in ministry up to her death. Their connections with other people kept these women active, vital, and engaged."

Happily, Dorothy's friends appreciate and understand her unique qualities. This has helped Dorothy manage the differences between what she perceived society expected of her and the life she chose to lead. "Go for it!" is her all-purpose advice. "I didn't finish college until I was 46 and had four children. I do what I can. Granted, at 77 I'm not planting 40,000 tree seedlings anymore, but I will put in 400 in March."

She wants to enjoy her life and age gracefully by taking time for the things that are really important. "I wish to keep my spontaneous sense of humor, my joy and laughter, and my emotional equilibrium. Without being morbid, I aim to stay in focus and to realize that I am *old*," she says. "I don't relate to appearance concerns because I have tried to have a healthy respect for who I am and how I am. I feel secure in myself. I'm not a worrier like some women. They are concerned about how they look, but I don't think about it because I think I look good."

It bothers her when she bumps up against societal stereotypes of older people. "A lot of us are still working and vital," she says. "We can be healthy and strong old people; we don't have to deteriorate."

. . . .

Ah, being young is beautiful,
but being old is comfortable.

. . . .

At the same time, Dorothy is philosophical. "My last day will come," says Dorothy calmly. "I am not supposed to be here forever. I'm resigned to the fact that it will all dissolve one day, sooner than I'd like." This may be part of what has increased her interest in religion lately. "I joined a Bible study group. We're all old ladies and we think alike."

Although women make up her most important friends, she does have a meaningful relationship with a man. "It's still possible to find one that is very rewarding," she says. "This relationship is not very different from my younger years. It's still a loving, caring relationship like I enjoyed with my husband."

Although she notes that many of her friends are not interested, she says, "We are sexual beings and I don't know if you ever lose that. I know I wouldn't want a relationship that wasn't sexual. No matter your age, you can keep a hot, burning passion for living large. There's still time."

Dorothy thinks than men and women fear aging equally, although they fear different things. "Men fear losing their macho image; women fear losing love," she says. "As friends and relatives die or move away, we must develop new relationships. These new people and their expectations of us will be different from any we have experienced previously." These new experiences help keep her young, she says.

Because Dorothy was a disciplined saver and investor throughout her career, she is in a good place financially. "I'm glad to have enough money to retire and do what I want," she says. She loves the opportunity that her position at the service agency provides for her to mentor and help so many women of all ages.

. . . .

WOMEN LIKE DOROTHY ARE REAPING the rewards of a good genetic inheritance combined with careful planning and a lifetime of good decisions. They enjoy good health and supportive relationships and use their talents well. When women expect to find adventure and newness they continue to learn and grow. Too many women are afraid of life. They worry about being alone or being sick and they have stopped living. Not Dorothy. She is planning for her future so she will not be a burden to others.

Not only is Dorothy taking the initiative, she has done the necessary homework to better understand her options including looking at assisted-living facilities to see what they are like. Even thought she does not like the idea she feels she must be prepared. She also has taken a really important step in her planning and she has discussed her thoughts with her children. Her children, however, see no reason for her to go to an assisted-living facility, saying they will make all the arrangements for her to stay with them. Dorothy is blessed with options and knows her children will care for her if and when the time comes that she is no longer able to care for herself. She intends, however, to be like the women who remained independent to the century mark, fully able to care for themselves.

Women like Dorothy have many strengths. Chief among these is a strong belief in self and the ability to remain independent. They are healthy and active. They have numerous friends and healthy relationships with their adult children. Many also see their sexuality as important and find satisfaction in a healthy male/female relationship. Although some women have given up hope of finding romance and sex because it seems unreachable, Dorothy wants to have it all. She mentors other women and coaches them about living fully in the moment.

Another reason Dorothy is successful with her own aging is that she has a belief in a higher power. Her belief systems tells her the day will come when she will leave this world and be rewarded with another life in a special place, so in many ways she looks forward to this reward. Dorothy is a planner. She would love for her health to remain as good as her mother's did into her nineties but she also is planning to be prepared should her health decline. Many of her friends are worried and fearful but she avoids this pitfall by planning and keeping lines of communication open with family and friends.

Dorothy is doing just fine and needs to keep doing what she's doing. She is a good role model for other women and she can share her experiences with others who worry about the future. Open communication seems to be one of the important keys to successful aging. Dorothy also has not fallen into the trap of stereotypical thinking about older women.

She admits she finds it frustrating that many in our society think that Seventies Women are old and incapable of living fully. She feels pretty lively! Her love life and her current love interest are a testimony for living, loving, and laughing more each year. She refuses to believe she has an expiration date and feels sad for women who believe their time is up and that it is time to move aside for younger women.

VIRGINIA: "I HAVE ENJOYED EVERY AGE — THEY HAVE ALL BEEN GOOD."

Virginia, 75, worries primarily about the health of her husband. He's ill and losing mental control, and she has set aside her own interests temporarily to take care of him. A former schoolteacher, horse trainer, and farm manager, Virginia has always been extremely capable and self-sufficient, yet she now faces the reality that she has entered a time of losses: of energy, of spouse, and of close friends. Death and illness have become an increasingly common — and depressing — topic of conversation in her circle.

"I'm not afraid of getting older, but long-term illness where there is no hope does scare me," she says. "I expected to be afraid," says Virginia. "Instead, I feel fortunate to have lived this long in good health. I have enjoyed every age — they have all been good. So I don't worry much."

Throughout her happy marriage and multiple careers, Virginia has taken time to consider the value of her life and to pursue her own interests. So when her husband is gone, as she expects he will be soon, she looks forward to getting back to them. "Life doesn't seem over to me," she says. Even so, she has faith in the dying process itself, and has overcome her fears about the end time by reactivating her faith. "I feel acceptance," she says. "Dying is just part of life."

Unlike Dorothy, who regarded her mother as an example of successful aging, Virginia says her mother "was a total queen and had a really hard time getting older." Her mother-in-law did much better. "She started writing a family history at 60, published it at 91, and died at 99. I try to emulate her by contributing what I can." Although Virginia has a full and active life, she hates what she sees in the mirror. Losing her youthful appearance has been hard for her to accept, and she had a tummy tuck a decade ago. "I always want to look terrific," says Virginia. "That means staying thin so I have tons of energy, and I keep up with the latest styles in clothing and hair." She tries every remedy she can find to stop her thinning hair and feels pleased when people say she doesn't look her age.

"When anyone asks me how old I am, my answer is always the same." Virginia says. "I say, 'That is really not a relevant question unless we are discussing examples of age discrimination.' Trust me, they never ask me again."

Virginia occasionally has trouble sleeping. When she asked her doctor for some advice and possibly medication, he said it was just a tough part of growing older that she needed to accept. Although this infuriated her, she didn't have the courage to confront him and express her feelings, and she admits that she worries about being dismissed by the medical community. When her request for a simple remedy was answered with such a negative, condescending view, she felt they were imposing a time limit on her being a healthy woman.

Virginia wants to retain her vitality and independence and says with a smile that her plan was always to keep charging hard until she died a sudden death at the same time as her husband. Since it looks now like he's going first, she is bracing herself for the loneliness of widowhood, but knows she, like so many of her friends, will survive it.

"As our abilities of body and mind diminish, some of our zest for life also decreases," Virginia points out. "We carry more baggage as we experience more difficulties and disappointments, and we become more boring to others as our interests narrow and we obsess about our health."

. . . .

I am a beautiful child of God.

. . . .

Continuing to learn and grow keeps Virginia's world from narrowing. "I have long considered myself a "work in progress" and I am constantly gathering vital information to assist me in my journey. I have found time to improve and magnify my natural talents and to discover new and fascinating areas of study." She had thought she'd be well over the hill by now, if not dead. Instead she finds herself still reasonably healthy, with many new interests in addition to her lifelong love of reading. In fact, getting older has brought her new gifts. "Even though I enjoy company, I am also quite comfortable by myself, unlike when I was younger."

Even though living expenses are always going up, Virginia thinks she and her husband will be OK financially. "I just hope I never have to ask our children for help," she says.

. . . .

VIRGINIA'S CHALLENGES REVOLVE AROUND HER husband's poor and declining health. It's no surprise that a husband's health has a direct correlation to a wife's health. Caregivers can and do develop health issues of their own if their partners' needs overwhelm them. Virginia has willingly accepted this job description for now and realizes that she has only limited time left with her husband. She is willing to set her personal interests aside.

Eighties Women who have lived a life full of health, fulfilling relationships, and a strong belief system often had positive role models. Women like Virginia's mother-in-law, now in her nineties, continue to be very successful role models and mentors. They show what it's like to live without fear of age, and without concerns for discrimination. Such women grow older while remaining strong and capable; they do not let the signs of physical aging diminish their self-confidence or feelings of self-worth.

Such successful models of aging help women to avoid feeling dismissed or invisible. In their roles as caregivers, women like Virginia are optimistic about their decisions to put the care of a spouse first. They are willing to wait for their own time, which will come soon enough. They have no intention of retiring from the world or from their friends and personal outlets but they see clearly what their priorities are for now.

In her turn, Virginia will be a good example for other women, a model of successful aging. Although her decision to put her husband first is a noble one, Virginia would do well to keep her own needs in mind lest she suffer ill effects due to stress and isolation while she cares for him. She needs to continue to stay present in the world as much as possible. Stress may catch up with a woman suddenly if she does not build respite into her days and find healthy outlets with her family and friends. She will probably find that her job as a full-time caregiver becomes more overwhelming after she has been doing it for a while. It is important for women to be sure to include activities that meet their own needs each day.

Now, before she feels overwhelmed, would be a good time for Virginia to find out what options are available in the community. Outreach services and support groups can help reduce feelings of isolation, grief, and the stress of full-time care. Dutiful caregivers often feel guilt as time passes and their spouses slowly fade and pass away. The void these women feel may be similar to what a mother experiences when she sends her last child off to school and faces her empty nest for the first time. At times like this it is good to have someone to help process these feelings.

BARBARA: "I'M THROUGH WITH MEN. I DON'T WANT TO TAKE CARE OF SOMEONE ELSE."

Barbara retired from her career as night nurse at a university health center at age 66. Now 79, she had received her LPN degree at age 40 and had raised four children. She has been married three times, divorced once, and was widowed twice.

"I never thought I'd live to be this age," Barbara says. "I'm through with men. I don't want to take care of someone else. We're all getting older, and I can handle my own problems but not someone else's."

Shortly after her third husband died, she suffered a serious accident that cost her a fourth of her brain. "I was changing a light bulb and received an electric shock. They didn't think I'd live, and I had to work really hard to come back. My mind works now.

"It's been good for me," Barbara says. "I don't take things for granted any more. I'm a little handicapped but I can live with that. In my heart I think I can get better. The generation I grew up in worked hard and I've overcome a lot. It's been slow and deliberate progress and I'm still working at it. It's a lifetime commitment."

She also experiences constant pain from fibromyalgia and arthritis. "But I can't sit and feel sorry for myself. If I just sit around it hurts worse and I get real stiff. So I stay active to keep my mind off it and try not to tell too many people.

Barbara knows she doesn't want to repeat her mother's life. "Mom never got out and walked. She used her heart murmur to justify a lot of resting and lived as a semi-invalid. My grandmother added to that. She lived with us and wanted to be useful. I don't think it was intentional, but by keeping my mother an invalid, Grandma could feel useful taking care of her daughter and the rest of us.

Barbara feels sad for older women who have to continue working because they don't have any money. "I lost half of my retirement at one time when the stock market went down." Despite those losses, she has enough to live comfortably if she is careful.

It didn't worry her to travel to another state to live in an apartment behind the house of her son and his wife. "I make my own decisions," she says. In time, however, her son's intensive travel schedule left her feeling lonely, and she moved back home where she had a broader support group. "It's nice to know my children love me and that they want the best for me. It may not always be what I want, but it's OK.

"After returning home I felt lonesome in my three-bedroom house. I knew the boys wanted to sell it because it was beginning to need lots of repairs." So she moved in with her daughter. "She works really hard cleaning houses and her husband is a truck driver who is gone a lot," Barbara says. "I try to keep up with my share. I do a little, then rest a little. I'm trying to keep her from getting ill because she also has fibromyalgia and lupus."

Living with her daughter took quite an adjustment. "I don't have any say about things, but I try not to make any waves." When her husband is home, "I try to do things in my room so I'm not under their feet," Barbara says. "We live pretty separately, although I may go to a show with them if they ask me. We just try to get along as best we can. One of the hardest times is when she's mad at me. I have to stand there and let her say it all; she gets upset with me if I walk off.

Barbara's first husband died. The second was an abusive alcoholic. "For 22 years I kept hoping he would change until I finally realized he would not. Part of what made me stay was that my mother thought divorce was the worst thing. One of the hardest things I ever did was to break with her and go ahead to do what I needed to do.

"Mom watched my sister dying by inches, living with an alcoholic. He attacked her all the time, especially toward the end when she got so disfigured with rheumatoid arthritis. After she died people told me that he went to the cemetery every day, but it was too late. My mom finally accepted that I had been right to leave and that it was for the best. Mom would babysit my kids, and we took on my niece and nephew."

Still, Barbara bears a burden of guilt for the example she set for her daughter. "I'm concerned about what I modeled for her. She drank a lot and worked in bars, but she is a good person.

"When you've been independent and worked all your life to survive, it's hard to give up your independence. Some women get hard after divorce and don't want to try again, but I remarried twice. Dealing with stepchildren takes a lot of communication, a lot of swallowing pride, and working things out with others," she says.

Barbara thinks that making other people happy is a key to a long life. "I just had cataracts removed from both of my eyes. A friend from church took me, and she loved to do it. She felt she was making me happy, which she was. And I was making her happy by allowing her to help me. Another friend of mine says she thinks she has lived so long because she does everything she can to help others," she says.

When she contemplates the end of her life, as Seventies Women tend to do with some regularity, Barbara says, "I just hope I don't have to suffer a long time; this is about the level of pain I can take. I take a muscle relaxant, a pain reliever, and an arthritis pill, and I'm not afraid of the possible heart attack side effects."

. . . .

BARBARA'S 30-YEAR UNIVERSITY CAREER HAS left her with reasonable financial resources in the form of both pension and savings plans. This financial base allows her to feel some security and to make decisions independently from her children. This is important to her self-image because she already struggles with her dependence on family members for emotional and physical contact. She feels at times that she is a burden and tries to compensate by helping in any way she can.

When a woman has a history of unsuccessful relationships she will worry if her example is now reflected in her own children's marriages and self-defeating behaviors. In addition to this emotional pain, Barbara has physical pain each day, which limits her energy and activities and further erodes her sense of control over her future. She fervently hopes her condition does not get worse because she feels that her daughter's health issues and her own are all they can handle.

One enduring strength women like Barbara possess is their ability to survive while maintaining optimism for the future. They have endured marriages and may have weathered years of abuse without becoming bitter or cynical. They have the love and support of their families even though their circumstances are sometimes painfully difficult. When they stay connected and try each day to remain active and helpful to their families and friends they can prevent any physical or emotional problems from getting them down. Barbara has learned to appreciate what she has and to reach out to help others; this enables her to wake each day with a purpose and to keep busy.

Because of the sporadic conflicts in her relationship with her daughter Barbara should find someone with whom she can openly and honestly discuss her living arrangements. Her children's lives appear to be somewhat chaotic and her own daughter appears to be headed toward more serious health problems. This may impose impossible burdens on a woman who is struggling with her own health. Women need to have a plan for long-term care that is independent from family members, especially if their situations are unstable. Barbara needs to put her own concerns first, at least until she has gathered information about long-term assisted-living arrangements and formulated and funded her plan. Her daughter's fragile physical and emotional health indicates it would be unwise for Barbara to build her plan for future care around her daughter's ability to help.

SHIRLEY: "THIS IS A DIFFERENT KIND OF AGING THAN I EXPECTED."

At age 75, Shirley has been a widow for 11 years. Her husband was sick for 13 years of their near-half-century marriage. "We had a good life together, and we worked together as a team. He was half of me, and in business we never competed with each other. We adopted two girls who were natural sisters, and now I have four lovely grandchildren. They are such a joy, and the relationship is good for them and good for me."

"I'm enjoying widowhood, but this is a different kind of aging than I expected," Shirley says. "I thought we would retire and travel. We kept putting things off, saying we'd do it later. It never happened.

"My mentor treated me like a friend. She listened and only gave advice when I asked for it, and sometimes not even then. She died at age 94, and she was a great role model of successful aging. Like her, I try to add something to every group I'm in," Shirley says. "I can sense people's needs and I make it my mission to get them to speak. It's my way of reaching out. Most people, if you sit down and talk to them and show some interest, you'll bring them out.

"The worst thing about aging would be losing my independence," she says. "That's why I'm building this house in town. I will be closer to my daughter who has a badly handicapped 8-year-old. I can help her out by picking up my grand-daughter. I will be closer to go to the beauty shop, the doctor, and the dentist, and I won't have to go out on a busy avenue to get groceries. My house on a golf course seemed too big and out of the way. I always wanted to do it and thought 'This is the time.' The move looms heavy, but I'll get it done."

Shirley accepts with calm all her life changes. "I'm not afraid of getting old and dying," she says. "I don't really want to be in a nursing home, but I've told the girls if I get dementia, then they have a right to do that. I have bought quite a bit of long-term care insurance to cover that.

"I do think women are underpaid," Shirley says. "Women should get equal pay for equal work. Our businesses were successful and I've been blessed to not have to worry about finances. That's why some women get married again." Shirley scorns the very idea, saying: "Most men are just wimps; they want someone to take care of them."

But there are disadvantages to being alone. "I sold my condo in Palm Springs last year because it's no fun to go by yourself. The man I was seeing would have liked to marry but I've got enough baggage with my children and their children; I don't want to take on someone else's.

"I miss the intimacy of sexual relationships but a big hug does us all a world of good," she says. Shirley's husband was on medication for years that made him impotent, but she says, "I never felt a lack of fulfillment. To me, just telling some-one you love them creates intimacy that fulfills me just as much."

She has learned to make do without male companionship, but: "The holidays are still hard, and I still don't like long weekends. I always want it to be Monday again." She has found that making plans helps her cope. "I go to brunch with a couple on Saturday mornings, then to church on Sunday. Then I break up the rest of the day when I go by and see my grandchildren. For a long time Sundays were bad days, but you just have to find or make your own way," she says.

Shirley is proud that she takes care of all her own business, and still drives to meet with her lawyer, stockbroker, and CPA. "I can't imagine not driving," she says. "Now that I've had my eyes done, I can see the road and the lines in the road and the cows up on the hill. What a beautiful world we have!"

. . . .

SHIRLEY'S CHALLENGES CENTER ON MAKING the remainder of her life feel worthwhile. Women like Shirley who have lived full lives running businesses and being independent see no reason to stop. Why should they? They want a new reason to get up each morning. Shirley's job changed when she stayed home to care for her sick husband whose health continued to fail and decline. Like so many other women, she took her job of caring for her husband very seriously even though society takes that role for granted. Day after day, a woman who is caring for someone else can find herself lower and lower on her list of important people and things. When the time came for Shirley to once again put her own needs upfront, it was a daunting and overwhelming task. Even today, Shirley feels most complete when she is busy helping or taking care of someone else.

Women like Shirley have so many strengths that have been honed through a lifetime of use. They are self-starters, highly motivated, and *very* proficient at caring for themselves. By now skilled at handling their own finances, they have what it takes to manage their everyday living and are confident about their self-care, at least for now. Shirley loves her independence and although she did have a satisfying relationship with a man after her husband died, she knows she does not want to take care of another man.

To meet their relationship needs, Seventies Women can stay connected to close friends and keep busy with their families. They love their grandchildren and feel good about helping their children cope; they are especially valuable when someone in the family has special needs. It is important that they have activities that let them feel capable and competent in this world. They know full well that as they grow older they will have to make adjustments even though they have done a lot of planning for the future. When they are fortunate enough to be financially stable they know they have been blessed with a good life. Their happiest future is filled with possibilities, friends, and family.

KEEPING YOUR MIND SHARP

. . . .

- ❧ Exercise and keep physically fit.
- ❧ Eat a diet rich in antioxidant fruits and vegetables and Omega 3 fatty acids.
- ❧ Get enough rest.
- ❧ Read, learn, and grow.
- ❧ Do routine things in a new and different way: Shower with your eyes shut; drive a new route home.
- ❧ Surround yourself with interesting people.
- ❧ Travel to experience new and exciting things.
- ❧ Do things that challenge you: learn a language, try a new job or skill.
- ❧ Volunteer and interact with others.
- ❧ Keep up with current events.
- ❧ Manage your stress level.

Shirley is doing well with her aging and she relishes her independence. The last thing a Seventies Woman wants is to be a burden to anyone. They much prefer relationships in which they can continue to take a helping role. However, they need to prepare themselves emotionally for a time when they may no longer be able to care for others or themselves. Shirley has not done this and the idea of asking for help from anyone depresses her.

A Seventies Woman who is well insured and financially capable of paying for any type of assisted living needs to consider where and what she wants. Once Shirley has investigated what is out there and planned her next move in various scenarios, she should discuss this with her family. She has become an integral part of her daughter's family and she might consider finding some other resources for them including possible financial assistance for the time when she is no longer there to help.

Even more importantly, though, Shirley needs to consider what she wants personally rather than taking on even more responsibility. These days belong to her and she has so much to give and to enjoy in her life. She may have another 15 to 20 years left and she is healthy and has no limits at this time. Shirley can do whatever she wants: Have some fun, travel, be a mentor, share her gifts, and be a good role model for other women. She has so much to share with other women about what it takes to be successful with aging in our society.

Staying independent is Shirley's greatest concern, so it's vitally important that she take time to exercise, eat well, and, of course, get regular checkups. Every Seventies Woman can benefit from talking with friends her own age about their challenges. They can all join forces and gain much support from one another.

WHAT DO SEVENTIES WOMEN WANT?

The stories of the Seventies Women (like those of Eighties Women to come) are some of the richest in experience and perspective of any women we spoke with. These women had a vast amount of knowledge and understanding of the world. Their looks were changing but not their desires to live a life with challenges, excitement, and relationships.

Seventies Women feel acutely the passage of time and focus increasingly on their awareness that life is infinitely precious. Three-fourths of Seventies Women say they do not fear aging. By now, they are familiar with the territory and much of the mystery is gone. Still, nearly 23 percent say they *are* afraid. Most of their fears relate to losing their health and independence. A great many Seventies Women also worry about their financial futures, now that they are contemplating the possibility of 15 to 20 more years and the possibility of needing long-term care.

They cope as best they can with the inescapable effects of the passing years, most of them with reasonably good humor. Most women were taught early in life that their physical appearance is their most important asset; some women never get over it. When normal aging takes their youthful glow, their self-esteem suffers. In a society that most values youth and beauty, some women punish themselves when advancing age robs them of their personal beauty. Virginia struggles to feel good about herself, despite her many fine qualities and overall wonderful life.

An older woman clearly cannot compete with the looks of youth, and 97 percent of Seventies Women have let it go; yet we found that three percent of women age 70 and older still rate their appearance as their most important aging issue. Seventies Women are not afraid to consider help from their plastic surgeon. Those who do often realize they have many years ahead. They want to look their best, so they think, "Why not take advantage of the miracles of modern medicine?"

Seventies Women Get It Together

If you don't see a good reason below to gather together with other women, make up your own.

🐾 Girlfriend getaways: to the city, country, spa, health club, or movies.

SEVENTIES WOMEN FEEL USEFUL WHEN THEY:

. . . .

* Help other people
* Make life easier for their kids
* Take care of their grandchildren
* Maintain their health
* Support their church
* Drive where they want
* Continue to broaden and nurture healthy relationships
* Check in with friends by telephone
* Visit shut-ins
* Continue to work to support themselves
* Volunteer
* Become mentors and role models for younger women
* Take on leadership roles
* Use their life experiences to help create positive changes

see sidebar next page

* Girls' night out — or in.
* Mentor women in your profession or the wider community.
* Find a mentor among the successful women in the community.
* Women's athletic clubs: bike, hike, swim, golf, work out, or play.
* Food-oriented groups: ethnic dinners, wine or coffee clubs, monthly lunch or dinner meetings.
* Political groups that educate women on the issues and help get out the vote.
* Hobby groups: Books, gardening, sewing, knitting, crafting, scrapbooking
* Faith group: Bible study, or study of world religions.
* Memory keepers: write memoirs, make books.
* Cards or board games.
* Philanthropic service groups: create donations for disaster victims (health kits of towel, washcloth, toothpaste, comb, soap); band together to help a friend or church member; support children or victims of domestic violence or the poor.

Nearly every woman 70 or older said a woman becomes old between the ages of 70 and 90. Most women in this age group have come to terms with the reality of their lost youth. In fact, they know they have much more serious challenges ahead: keeping their good health and their independence and the energy to care for themselves. Their wishes for themselves reflect their differing personalities.

Women who feel invisible talk honestly about their frustrations with growing older and how a society that is youth-driven ignores and devalues women as they age. Having positive and healthy female role models seems to be the best factor in predicting whether or not a woman will age successfully. Women without good role models more often internalize the negative views society projects onto aging persons in the United States, particularly onto aging women.

With their acute sense of passing time, many say wistfully, "I wish I had more time," "I wish I had a way to go visit loved ones and friends," and "I wish I could stay as healthy as I am now."

FEELING GOOD ABOUT SEVENTIES LIFE

By their seventies and beyond, women are really counting the years and trying to predict how their self-care abilities will endure, not just in the physical realm, but financially and emotionally as well. They know the importance of good support systems and more than ever are beginning to look realistically at the big picture of caring for themselves as they grow older.

Having positive role models seems to help women feel good about themselves as they get older. Some seem to sail through aging and continue to feel successful and productive throughout their advancing years. Not surprisingly, having seen other women maximize the positive aspects of growing older seems to make them more able to envision a positive experience for themselves. Some women also channel their personal power, passion, and feeling of accomplishment to help other women and create positive changes in their communities.

The upbeat realism of the comments of these Seventies Women makes clear that any age can be good as long as a woman retains joy, love, laugh-

SEVENTIES WOMEN FEEL USEFUL WHEN THEY:

- ❀ Run for a public office
- ❀ Help other women enter into politics
- ❀ Make their votes count

One of the many things no one tells you about aging is that it is such a nice change from being young.

MAINTAINING HEALTHY RELATIONSHIPS

. . . .

- ❦ Consider being a role model and leader for younger women.
- ❦ Share your experiences from your work, career, or hobbies—do not let all of those life experiences go and be wasted.
- ❦ Keep a good sense of humor and find laughs wherever you are.
- ❦ Maintain curiosity about others and about life.

ter, compassion, and empathy for others. These women have served as mentors and pioneers for other women in their peer group. Women who do not accept the stereotypes of aging continue to feel successful as they seek their bliss and passion in the world. These women have placed themselves in the use-it-or-lose-it camp and they absolutely intend to wear out, not rust out.

By observing women in their seventies, we can gain a phenomenal understanding of how women succeed at aging. Their example helps women understand that neither changes in physical appearance nor age itself needs to sideline a woman; instead, we can stay in the game and have full and exciting lives throughout our later years. Remember Grandma Moses? She began painting in her eighties. Some Seventies Women may have just received their "marching orders," so the world had better watch out! It also is OK to be sexy and to want it all. Seventies women are not quiet about any of this and many of these women expect to live a long life with a lot of loving, laughing, and living. And why not?

Many Seventies Women find that their interest in spiritual matters increases. As they come to terms with aging, changing bodies, and flagging energy, they become acutely aware that their time is running short. If they have not previously found comfort in spirituality, many begin to search harder, seeking ways to cope with their mortality. Women who find faith and strength from a higher power also discover they grow in self-confidence and hope for their futures. They are amazed to feel their fears diminish and to enjoy a new sense of freedom.

I think we are aging our whole lives. A woman isn't old until she decides to be.

Although many Seventies Women seem to have outgrown their fear of aging, a woman's basic temperament (her optimism or pessimism) probably remains reasonably consistent throughout her lifetime. While some women ruminate over their regrets, others seize what time they still have available to make every possible life dream come true. The woman who has taken the time to consider the value of her life and who uses her remaining time to pursue her interests seems best prepared to enjoy her old age. At the other extreme, the woman who has remained in denial and let age catch her by surprise is often frustrated by regrets and "woulda, coulda, shoulda's." Growing and learning each day is clearly a key to living longer, healthier lives, and achieving the greatest joy.

BETTER CARE FOR MYSELF

Women of any age who seek passion both emotionally and physically can find love and romance no matter what their ages might be. Coming to terms with changing relationships is a major developmental task for Seventies Women as they grow older. Many have voluntarily stepped out of relationships with men, whom they seem to view as dependent, needy, and demanding. This was much less true for Sixties Women and may reflect a change in gender roles and expectations. Men — and women — born before World War II may have assumed that caretaking was a female's lot.

SEVENTIES WOMEN WANT OTHERS TO KNOW

- ❀ I want my family to stop worrying about me so much. I can take care of myself.
- ❀ I am a capable and responsible human being. Do not discount me.
- ❀ I hate to ask for help. It makes me feel weak and incompetent.
- ❀ I want to keep good relationships with my friends and family; I need that support and connection.
- ❀ I worry about managing my money and other affairs by myself.
- ❀ I want to be respected and heard as a mature and intelligent person.
- ❀ I have much to offer and I intend to live a long and productive life.

see sidebar next page

SEVENTIES WOMEN WANT OTHERS TO KNOW

. . . .

- ❀ I want my children to see me as still capable (yet be willing to help me later).
- ❀ I have worked hard and planned carefully to get where I am today.

Life itself is change, and acceptance and understanding of this fact helps ease the aging process. Seventies Women have experienced many changes: husbands or partners die, energy and health fade, and close friends and family members die or move away. As in other areas of aging, women who have gained knowledge and skills, and enjoyed role models and mentors who took these changes in stride are more likely to feel successful. Many women report they truly enjoy their peaceful solitude and relish taking care of only themselves for the first time in their lives. This is good, because the majority live without a partner. In every census from 1970 to 2000, about three-fourths of women aged 65 and older lived alone. In contrast, about one-fifth of men aged 65 and older lived alone.

Of women between the ages of 75 and 84, one-third are married and still living with a spouse. More than half are widows. About one in ten either never married or has divorced. Not surprisingly, widows as a whole had the least confidence of Seventies Women in their ability to take care of themselves in the coming years. While this probably relates to their age, it may also reflect a lack of insurance and savings to provide resources they could use to care for themselves.

Seventies Women also now focus more and more on their concerns for future generations. They watch with pride as their adult children, nieces, or nephews take up the baton of life, or they watch with regret and consternation as they fail. Either way, no one wants to be a burden to the next generation. Often older women continue to make an invaluable contribution to their families with their additional income, their labor, and with daily care for children and grandchildren.

Although most Seventies Women are still strong and energetic, chronic illnesses take an increasing toll; even those who practice the best of self-care will have bad days. Many women have a touch of arthritis. Others have joint replacement, a broken bone, digestive complaints, fading vision, muscle weakness and, of course, pain.

Finding the right doctor to listen and to help with their aging issues is a concern for many older women. Although many women talk in general terms about their health, few identified concerns about the major health concerns that kill or cripple women, such as heart disease, cancer, and diabetes. The typical woman may be overly concerned for her family's well-being and overlook her own. Here are the top three reasons women ignore their health: 1) My doctor didn't say anything about it. 2) He said it's all in my head. 3) It's just part of aging; I'll get used to it.

A nursing home administrator commented that most of the rural women who enter nursing homes are destitute, meaning Medicaid funds their stay. Even so, the administrator says they love it and are so happy because for the first time someone is doing something for them; they have basically lived as slaves their whole lives.

NORMAL AGE-RELATED MEMORY LOSS OR DEMENTIA?

Normal age-related memory loss	Dementia
Forgetting names you remember later	Memory gaps that impair daily living
Forgetfulness stays about the same	Forgetfulness gets worse
Forgetting words	Forgetting how to do things you've done many times before
Forgetting the name of a blender	Forgetting how to use a blender
Telling someone a story again	Repeating phrases or stories in the same conversation
Did I pay that bill?	Difficulty handling choices or money
Slower to learn new things	Can't learn new things
What did I come into this room for?	Doing things that require steps, like a recipe
Forgetting which day you did something.	Losing track of what happens each day

EMOTIONS OF SEVENTIES WOMEN

. . . .

- ❧ Concern that time is running out
- ❧ Desire to make the most of life
- ❧ Cherishing relationships with close friends and family
- ❧ Connecting spiritually with self
- ❧ Worrying about health and self care
- ❧ Fear of being a burden to others
- ❧ Sadness about body changes and physical limitations
- ❧ Wondering if their savings will last their lifetimes
- ❧ Striving to perform at work and avoid being passed over
- ❧ Desire to be seen as capable of important thoughts
- ❧ Fear of becoming invisible and being dismissed by others

see sidebar next page

Why are women ignoring their own health instead of seeking out prevention and early treatment for diseases? What is happening to women after these years and are they getting the medical interventions needed for diagnosis and treatment early in the disease process?

Besides, what seems to most worry so many women is not so much a disease, disorder, or change in their physical, psychological, or emotional status, as the prospect of being a burden and not being able to care for themselves. One must wonder if most of these women have *ever* had a good experience of being cared for. In truth, most probably have not. One of the greatest things Seventies Women can model for later generations is good self-care. If women can learn to truly take care of themselves and not to ignore or deny health issues, they would reap the reward of catching problems early and enjoying better overall health.

NEEDING A MONEY PLAN

Half of all women over age 65 live on less than $12,000 a year; half of men live on less than $20,000. Small wonder that finances are a major concern for women of all ages. Many women have primary responsibility for family finances and spend their entire lives trying to make ends meet. Unable to get more education to get a better job, they arrive at retirement underfunded and unprepared. Women who have depended on a man for support have a different type of problem when the man disappears through death or divorce. Typically, women's income drops sharply after divorce.

Women who have let their husbands handle everything must learn to pay the bills, pull their lives together, and support themselves. They often discover their small incomes require them to work for several more years. Fortunately, Medicare and Social Security provide a safety net, although it's a net with a lot of holes. Women who have improved their earning ability and done effective financial planning can act as mentors for younger women to help them provide for their own financial security. As Seventies Women know so well, Prince Charming may not show up, and every women needs to prepare herself for that likelihood.

STILL FEELING YOUTHFUL

Most women aged 70 and beyond are realists who have found hope and satisfaction in their lives and have learned to enjoy each day. They have let go of trying to fit into society and worrying what it thinks about them. Many women scoff at what society says they should do, be, or think as they grow older. Independent women like this find their place in society, if they did not know it already, by following their instincts and picking up activities that matter to them. For example, nearly seven percent of Peace Corps volunteers are age 50 or older.

"I was more or less told that once I hit 40 it was time to put away bright colors, get a pair of dumpy shoes, and wear my hair in a conservative bun," said Dorothy's cousin Marge. "That is a bunch of baloney. I keep doing what I want to and saying what I want to and I am doing just fine." At 75,

EMOTIONS OF SEVENTIES WOMEN

- Happiness to express own feelings without worrying about the good opinion of others
- Feeling satisfied and relaxed
- Comfortable drawing on life experiences to help with each day

Marge advocates for women, and has helped many younger women move beyond female stereotypes as they grow older and wiser.

Women like Virginia seem to age more successfully because they have been able to find good role models and mentors. It's that recurring theme: women of all ages seek — and find — answers from other women who have been successful in getting this aging thing down and living long and productive lives. Seventies Women make clear that wanting to feel energetic and vital despite the advancing years is a universal desire — and challenge. Many women are pleased to be able to say, "Worry about aging? Not me! I'm too busy to care."

A woman who feels like she is the only one with this problem, and that everyone else is doing better with it than she is, needs to get out and talk more with other women. When women truly feel safe and let down their hair and tell the truth, they get *really* serious. The ones who feel scared and unprepared can learn a lot from the ones who don't seem to have much trouble. Those who have an attitude of gratitude find they can be thankful for the life they have and the people they have in it.

Dr. Nancy's Kick-Butt Keys for Seventies Women

- Challenge yourself to learn something new each day.
- Get a pet to love that you can hug.
- Find a creative outlet for your emotions and feelings, such as painting, sculpture, writing, or learning to play the piano.
- Eat well, exercise regularly, and get plenty of rest.
- Understand your budget and how to live within it.
- Abandon worry and resentment and embrace faith.
- Adopt a positive attitude rather than ruminating about problems.
- Understand that your worth doesn't really change with age.
- Be realistic in your expectations of yourself and others.

With so much energy, excitement, strength, and support among Seventies Women, what might we expect from Eighties Women? Although their numbers are dwindling, we find so many who are full of life, opportunities, and interest in what's coming around the bend. Many Eighties Women are just beginning to plan their next adventure.

As women grow older, many reject the limits they had put on themselves, as well as the limits they allowed others to impose. Freedom for many women comes later in life. For this they are glad and so are we. Many know they may have another 20 years of life and are starting to say "when I have my one-hundredth birthday I am going to do or be: _____. Women can choose from a universe of options to fill in that blank.

Visit www.womenspeak.com to learn more about the seventies. Express yourself and share ways you have learned, grown, and found your best life.

CHAPTER 8

The **8O**s
*Older, Savoring Life
and Pursuing Happiness*

*This aging thing is not what I had feared; the best part
is I say what I want and do what I want.*

PHYLLIS, 88

A woman who celebrates her eighty-first birthday today can expect to live at least nine more years to become 90. Many will live much longer. Eighties Women are usually surprised to find themselves this old. Even those who expected to live into their nineties think, "I can't be this close *already*!" Born before telephones and automobiles were widely used, they marvel at the changes in technology that they have witnessed. Equally amazing are the societal changes: women had few options and did not even win the right to vote until 1920.

WHAT EIGHTIES WOMEN WORRY ABOUT

Their life experiences have rendered Eighties Women more philosophical than younger women about human nature, about the course of life, and about their own limitations. Sorrow in all its forms — for the loss of spouses, friends, children, and youth — has softened their perspective into an appreciation of each day. Still, they are annoyed to be ignored, unafraid of speaking their minds, and retain their zest for life and friends. These wonderfully self-reliant women express a hesitancy to discuss their very personal issues. Many report they were taught to not discuss problems or concerns in public; it was considered to be improper behavior and poor manners. Many even blush when they talk about physical concerns.

These survivors have passed the normal life expectancy dictated by the actuarial tables yet are still going strong. They feel most successful in these advanced years when they stay connected with friends and family to avoid isolation and retain their support. If they can keep stretching themselves and avoid surrendering to fears, they continue to have new experiences to attract their interest and make them interesting to others. Those who continue to find ways to contribute to others and to improve their world through church or politics or other service derive great satisfaction from feeling useful. For them, hard work is the expected norm and all of these women have a strong work ethic in addition to their concern for others, and they often give little thought to their own needs.

In this chapter Mildred, Nora, Doris, and Helen show us through their composite profiles that Eighties Women can still feel as youthful, excited, and alive as women in their thirties. Of course, they dislike the physical effects of aging, but the most successful ones push themselves to stay as active, vibrant, and connected as possible. Their interest in life is as strong as ever and they provide invaluable support for their families and friends. Their example and inspiration provides an excellent role model for younger women.

MILDRED: "MY GREATEST BLESSING IS THAT I HAVE TO WORK."

Mildred, 81, had a happy 45-year marriage during which she performed several jobs. She worked as a meat cutter, then together with her husband she managed a hotel and later a small-town funeral home. He died 15 years ago. He didn't believe in insurance and they didn't have much put away. Now she has moved to a larger town where she still works as a realtor, a field in which an older woman can still successfully compete.

"Younger realtors will listen when I give advice, even though we're in hot competition with each other," she says. In return for her advice, the younger women help her with the new technologies and gadgets that have transformed the world of real estate like so many others. In truth, her biggest concern is what will happen when she can't work anymore.

Although she tries to approach life with a positive attitude, the prospect for getting really old frankly scares her. In her day, it was considered normal for the husband to handle all money issues. "I do worry about my financial ignorance, because I'm trying to get my affairs, assets, and belongings in order so it will not be a problem for my children," she says.

Mildred worries a lot: about terrorism, about violence in the schools, avoiding the complications of diabetes and hypertension, about her appearance, about having enough energy to keep up with her house, about what people think of her, and that her sons might die — or be killed — before her. "Most of all I fear being physically dependent or mentally incompetent," she says. Her father died a horrific death from dementia (probably Alzheimer's disease) and she worries about losing her mental and emotional well-being. Whenever she has trouble remembering something, she is sure that she is developing Alzheimer's as well.

"My mother, who was well-educated and strong, unfortunately fell into isolation and martyrdom," Mildred says. "She did not have much happiness in her old age." Mildred notices her own tendency to play the martyr and tries hard to avoid the victim mentality, yet she finds it hard to break habits that were passed down to her from mother. Like so many women her age, Mildred wishes she'd had more positive role models to demonstrate successful aging. Women her own age do not discuss their aging concerns openly and this often leaves her feeling alone and isolated with her anxieties.

Mildred used to love to turn heads, but that ended three decades ago. She tries to be philosophical. "I do miss my good appearance," she says. "The things I like least are the hanging jowls, the drooping facial skin. I color my hair but I can't do too much about wrinkles except smile, and hope they notice the dimples and not the wrinkles." She worries more about presenting an image of vitality than beauty, and only feels invisible when her energy and attitude are especially low. "But it is true that older women are invisible to many men," she notes. When she yearns for male companionship, she tells herself that is not likely. "It's just a dream."

If she had one wish, it would be, "To have my spouse alive so he would reassure me that he loves me no matter how old I look." Although she knows it is impossible she also daydreams — like most fearful women of every age — about going back in time 20 years. This magical number seems to signify a time when they felt strong, beautiful, and capable.

. . . .

*I never intended to get old, I was
just too busy. What the heck, I am not old.*

. . . .

Even women like Mildred who are afraid of getting older still perceive much sweetness in their lives. "Probably my greatest blessing is that I have to work," says Mildred. "This has forced me to continue to grow, improve, keep my health, and stretch my abilities. Keeping a schedule is important, because when I have to get up and get someplace, I tend more to my appearance. I am aware that I need much more rest than I used to, so I leave work to take a nap every day. And I make time to do something fun, either alone or with a friend, or talk with my best friend or my big brother. I enjoy life."

Mildred hopes she offers to those who see her a positive example of an older woman surpassing society's expectations of older women. Being still able to work and take care of herself makes her feel vital and competent. And she still has high hopes.

"I feel my time growing short with much left to do," she says. "I want to take trips, socialize with friends and family, improve my home and garden, read. I try not to think about it, but old age is hell and the worst years are still ahead." Her realistic assessment does not impair her overall positive attitude, however, and Mildred retains a sense of hope about her remaining days and tries to use each one wisely.

Mildred recognizes that an older woman's relationships will not necessarily always involve a male partner. "As a woman matures she should become more tolerant, patient, understanding, forgiving, and loving," Mildred says. "An older woman really needs reassurance that her family members and friends will be supportive. When younger family members have to become more helpful, they in turn enjoy being appreciated more." Others take for granted that their children will help them, just as they have helped the previous generation. "When I was in my thirties," recalls Mildred, "my mother-in-law had a stroke and came to live with us. This became somewhat of a problem as we moved several times with my husband's work and our family expanded." Still, she did not resent the responsibility, and Mildred expects her son, in his turn, to do the same. Mildred understands that this is a rite of passage and that others will take care of her, just as she has taken care of others who could no longer care for themselves.

"My son flies for a parcel delivery service so he travels all the time. He's building a duplex patio home so I can live in one side." Mildred is one of the millions of seniors who are lucky enough to have family support and assurance they will be cared for when they no longer are able. "I'm proud to see that my children are caring and thoughtful and concerned about others rather than focusing on their clothes and other material things," she said. "Humanity is their way of life."

Although she is pleased with the support she feels from her children, the lack of consideration from other members of society annoys her. Fortunately, she still feels able to control this part of her life. "It makes me mad that my doctor comes into the office late. Since I'm due to get the access-a-ride bus to go home soon after, I feel rushed during our appointment," says Mildred. "This is something I need to change."

Mildred is one of the few women over eighty who is still working. "I make good money but I don't have much cushion, so I am concerned about surprises ... negative ones. I'm afraid that should I have to stop working, there will not be enough money," she says.

Beauty is important to Mildred in all aspects of her life. She has put much energy and money into making a beautiful home. She enjoys using shells and beads to make beautiful jewelry. Yet she knows that age steals beauty from a woman. "It would be easier to age comfortably if society accepted women's value at all ages and placed less stress on appearance and beauty," she says. She sees a few rays of hope in the form of slowly changing social attitudes and greater awareness of women's needs as they grow older. This gives her some comfort and hope for women's futures.

. . . .

LIKE SO MANY WOMEN IN our society, Mildred struggles against feeling that age has stolen her place in society. The marks of the years on her face and body announce to the world that she has arrived in that foreign and often misunderstood place, old age. Because she has had no mentor or role model to show her how to age successfully, she is making it up as she goes along.

When women like Mildred are able — finally — to share her worries and concerns openly, they are surprised at the feelings of release and calm they experience. If more women would talk honestly about aging, they might find it less frightening. Being cared for by one's children is something many mature, capable women dread but, in fact, Mildred is one of the lucky ones in that her son expects to help her. Women who can plan with family members and talk about it openly can come to terms with the possibility and are less likely to feel shocked and powerless when they do need their children's help.

Mildred's lack of financial awareness puts her at a real disadvantage. Like so many women, she allowed her husband to take care of everything and was caught unprepared by his death. Death and divorce are the two scenarios that shock many women into dealing for the first time with bills, a shrinking reserve, and no dollars for long-term care and medical issues. Like so many other women, Mildred has no pension to augment her Social Security, so she must work as long as she can to try and catch up. The hardest part is that this is happening at a time that she feels her energy lessening and feels less drive to compete with younger men and women in the real estate market.

Mildred feels some regret that she has not better prepared herself financially, yet she is not letting her regrets immobilize her. She knows that regret is a waste of her precious time and energy, so she's trying to channel those feelings into talking with her children about being prepared and trying to model the behaviors of successful aging. She finds that it helps to talk with her friends and knows she is not alone in feeling unprepared. If her own mother had talked about her aging concerns, worries, and fears, Mildred thinks she would have been forewarned.

Women who know what their strengths are and who use them to their best ability often actually feel energized by the challenges they face. The lucky ones have support from their families; even if they have few financial resources to pay for long-term care, their children include them in their plans. Living in one side of her son's patio home will allow Mildred to preserve her independence while living in the context of a family that loves and supports her.

Mildred is alive and involved. Staying active and making each day count helps keep Eighties Women youthful in spirit and in mind. These lucky women get up, dress for the day, and renew their determination to make a difference in each one. They stay connected with work, community, and family and see the importance of sharing their experiences with others. All of these behaviors help women remain healthy and active.

Women like Mildred are doing well by all accounts. They use their smiles to win the hearts of others and try out new strategies to feel young, alive, and visible to co-workers, clients, and the world. They have good communication skills and know that both staying connected and keeping up with change are critical to success.

Mildred also knows she has to take responsibility for her finances. That's good, because it is never too late to learn. Taking control of this process helps women feel more aware and in control of their lives. The more decisions they can make about the future, the more comfortable they will be if they become physically, emotionally, or mentally unable to make decisions for themselves. All women wonder how other women their age are doing with their plans, and they feel better when they share their experiences. Even though Mildred is fearful about her future, she is talking about it and looking for commonsense solutions to assist her with these issues.

NORA: "WHAT IS YOUR FACE DOING FOR YOU? IT MAY BE TIME TO UPDATE."

Nora, age 86, has never accepted aging and for nearly 60 years has celebrated an annual "unbirthday." Although she claims she "never thought about aging," she has consistently concealed her age and had a facelift in her fifties. "I always expected to live into my nineties. "I don't feel old in my mind — just middle-aged. I take as good care of myself as I can. I exercise three times a week, walk the dog, keep moving, and always take my vitamins. My kids grew up seeing me in front of the TV exercising to Jack LaLanne and they would follow along with my exercise routine."

Nora moved 10 years ago to her younger daughter's community, which had also been Nora's childhood home. Where she lived before, no one had known her age (due to the unbirthdays), but with this move, people remember her from high school and college and can identify her age.

Nora thinks that people who struggle with aging have an inferiority complex that robs them of confidence in self and their ability to take action. They think they're not pretty, or their clothes don't fit, or they can't talk to people, whatever. It interferes with their view of self. "Age means nothing to me; it's better than the alternative," she says. "I'm not afraid and I'm not thinking about *getting* old — I *am* old. Actually I prefer to use the word *mature*. I figure it's amazing that I got this far so whatever I'm doing is OK."

"This last year I've really known I'm 86. I can't hit a golf ball as far as I used to. Little things creep up, like my voice is changing. A friend on the phone said, "What's the matter with your voice? It sounds old." She sometimes feels defensive and says, apologetically, "I never meant to get old." But then she stops herself and says, "I am not *old*, I am just *older*." Nora admits she had expected to be able to keep doing everything she had always done, so she feels her body has let her down and sometimes she feels sad about that.

Caring for her husband, who is losing ground to Alzheimer's disease, is an increasing strain on Nora. "Relationships change and you adjust," she says. "But I'm not overwhelmed with it yet. It's natural to have good days and bad days. I just live one day at a time and don't dwell on it. And I pray a lot." She has watched so many of her friends struggle with the loss of their husbands that she does not look forward at all to being alone. Many days when she feels tired, she just reminds herself that she must keep going to be sure her husband is cared for. She sees this as her job and it keeps her going.

"I'm just too busy to accept being old. When I look in the mirror and see wrinkles I think, I earned every one. Age is a state of mind and we all do it." That said, Nora keeps looking in the mirror to see what she might want to "update" next. Her recommendations: "Ask yourself, 'What is your face doing for you?'" and "Keep a good relationship with your plastic surgeon." Nora is one of a growing number of ordinary women who see nothing wrong with a little help from their doctors.

"When I was a child we moved a lot," Nora says. Her father was always being transferred to sell for another feed mill. "Times were tough and I remember Daddy worrying and talking with Mother about the Depression.

"My mother was a good role model for aging," says Nora. "Mom was an outspoken, strong lady even though she was only 5-feet 2-inches tall. She was so busy during the Depression. We knew it was tough but at Christmas time each of us had lots of presents to open. It might just be a pair of socks, or some other little thing that was important to us. She did it all and I never felt poor. She stayed sharp in her mind until she died and never ever complained or worried about getting older. She lived to be 94."

Nora graduated from college in 1944 with a degree in chemistry and biology and went to work in the lab of a big military hospital. "We had 5,000 beds during the war. They tried to hire me to replace the chief tech, but I knew the salary range and refused their offer. The new hire started out making so much less than the man who had just quit. We were aware of those things throughout our careers. The glass ceiling is still there. Although some have managed to break through, they're more the exception than the rule.

"I married in 1948, and had two children," Nora recalls. "My husband was an alcoholic who died when we were both 52 and the kids were in high school. He committed suicide. What a selfish act! He was not thinking of anyone but himself.

"My mom never even finished high school but she was behind us every step of the way. She got all three of us to go to college. She used to say, 'I wish I knew how to do something so I could work, too', but Daddy didn't want her to. Everything they did encouraged us to want to do well. From the minute we graduated from college, not one of us ever took a penny from Mother and Daddy."

Nora has always had a fear of being a burden, and still really wants to stay independent. "I have a torn rotator cuff that needs surgery, so I will be dependent on people for a while, but that's only temporary," she says. "The best thing when you get older is holding onto your health to be physically well so you can keep yourself going. A lot of it is due to your genes; I've tried to take care of myself because both sides of my family lived to be very old.

"I'm concerned about having to stop driving. I love to get in my car and if I have to give up my keys I'll feel isolated. My kids say 'Don't worry — we'll pick you up.' But I don't want to call for every little thing. I *won't*.

"So many older women say they feel devalued," Nora says. "I think they feel left out in social ways, or their own families are no longer interested or paying attention. It's not that they don't value us. They just don't regard us as interesting. At big family dinners I occasionally think, 'I wish someone would ask what *I* think.'"

That's why she thinks it's especially important to have her women friends. "We're all interested in what the others are doing," she says. "Younger people don't relate to our past like our friends do. My cousin moved to Hawaii with her husband, going somewhere she did not have a single friend. What a mistake! I would be really lost without my friends. It's great to get out and have fun. I always make time for my friends."

With the advancing years, Nora has suffered many losses. "We were once eight in my bridge club, now we are just three. I've just had a third friend kill herself. One had severe depression; the second had a Valium addiction, divorce, and a psychiatric illness; the third one thought her cancer had recurred and she gave up. We've all learned to be a little kinder to each other and not so judgmental," Nora says. "You can't know what other people are thinking."

....

I intend to keep driving and going to Curves.
When I'm one hundred I hope they throw me
a surprise birthday party. At the least, I would
love to hear from Today Show host Willard
Scott (that is, if he is still alive!) Janet, 82

....

She thinks women are lucky to have a girlfriend network. "Men don't so much call to chat on the phone and say 'Let's go to lunch,'" Nora observes. "I think that's why when they're old, they're so much more alone.

"I have four children, all very smart. They take after their mother," Nora says with a twinkle. "I'm close to the kids, and national politics interest me partly because of my concern for the future for my grandchildren who are growing up in a tough time. Grandchildren are such a joy," she says. "Looking back, I wish that instead of cleaning the house, I had spent time more with my children."

As Nora struggles with her surprise and wonder about her reality as an Eighties Woman, she has no more room for denial or excuses about her changing appearance, wrinkles and all. She is face to face with what were distant worries for her as a younger woman. Her low energy and changed physical strength and endurance have left Nora frustrated with her inability to move and function as she once did. Continuing to be able to drive and keep her independence are her key issues. Nora has only grudgingly given up her beloved game of golf and she fears the day when she must also give up driving.

Although she worries about losing car privileges, Nora's biggest challenge may be that she is the primary caregiver for her husband with Alzheimer's disease. Research shows that when a person with Alzheimer's is hospitalized or dies, their spouse faces a greatly increased risk of death. Many loyal, loving women like Nora see this as their ultimate responsibility; the burden is theirs to keep. Although they do not resent the job, they do worry about being alone when their spouse is gone. Many Eighties Women also find it difficult to ask for help, which leaves them in a risky position for their own declining physical, emotional, and mental health and they often feel isolated.

Among Nora's many strengths is the fact that she is dealing with her aging concerns in a primarily healthy fashion. Although many women are surprised by their own — and the world's — reactions to their visibly aging appearance, for the most part they realistically accept this as a natural process. None of them like the way society views the aging woman, but they do understand it and deal with it by staying busy and active and involved with friends and family.

However, women who are caregivers really need to take more time for themselves and place "Take care of me" higher on their to-do lists. They need a better understanding, both of the stress they experience when constantly caring for a spouse, and of the implications this stress has for their own health. Their husbands will inevitably continue to lose ground and they must prepare themselves for the day when they are no longer able to manage alone. Finding resources now is a top priority, and the nearest Alzheimer's Association office is a great place to start. These associations have many services for both patients and their families and support groups help family members learn to deal with losing a person day by day to Alzheimer's.

Nora's health and continued mobility has to be a top priority for her and her family. In-home healthcare aides can help a lot and can be part of a back-up plan if something should happen to her. This is where children and families must be invited into the discussion. Eighties Women would do well to make decisions now, with their children involved, so they will know and understand their parents' wishes should they become unable to care for themselves.

When women stay connected with friends in church and community groups, they can maintain an active social life. This definitely requires that they develop alternative forms of transportation. Driving at night or in unfamiliar parts of town are already problems for many Eighties Women, so lining up reliable help and transportation now will save stress and confinement later should they become unable to drive.

DORIS: "FAMILIES DIDN'T USED TO TALK MUCH TO THEIR DAUGHTERS ABOUT THE UPS AND DOWNS OF LIFE."

Doris, age 89, had four brothers. "I was the only girl and they named me after the midwife who delivered me into this world. I've had a good life. I was born in a tiny rural town where they still go back on Memorial Day to the old cemetery. We were very poor. My mentor was my schoolteacher, who taught the whole family in a one-room school. She told me I could be anything and I always kept this in the back of my mind. I grew up during the Depression."

She wanted to go to beauty school but her family did not have enough money. "So I got a job as a sales clerk," she says. "I married and had a child before my husband went to war, but when he returned he was a changed person. It didn't work out. After I found out I had cancer, I got a divorce. I thought 'I'm going to have to take care of myself and my son, so I can't take care of you, too.'"

Her second husband passed away seven years ago after being ill for five years. "When it was over I had no guilt although I missed him terribly," she recalls. "The loneliness when you are first widowed is god-awful and you think you'll never get over but you do. You adjust.

"I never let my wrinkles bother me," says Doris. "I would never consider a facelift anyway; I've seen too many that are not a good thing. God put me here with what I have to take care of as best I can. When you visit with people you hardly notice their looks, anyway — unless it's outstanding, and even then there are other things to pay attention to. Overweight must be hard, though," she says thoughtfully. "Some people can't seem to handle their bodies.

"Younger women need to realize that good health and energy give you more power; they need to take care of themselves. Even if you have physical problems, life can still be good if you have your mind," Doris observes, noting that, "If your back goes out on you, there's less energy for healing than when you're 30."

Although she's in perfect health without an ache or pain (she walks and does Pilates exercises daily, runs several times a week, and enjoys participating in walk/run benefit activities) she thinks at 89 the odds are she might not live much longer. "Maybe I should move out of this big house and settle everything so my grandkids would get what I want," she says. "But then the kids come home for Thanksgiving and Christmas and I think, 'Oh, I'll just let the kids take care of it later.'"

Doris stays close to her family. "I'm never too busy to do something for them," she says. "They think I'll never get old. I'm 89, but I still drive."

When Doris was growing up, families did not talk to their daughters about the ups and downs of life, she says. "My mother and I never discussed anything like this. When I was growing up, if you had a problem you just dealt with it yourself and moved on. I was never allowed to be sad or worried about anything.

My mother would just say, 'Look on the sunny side of life,' or 'There are so many other people with bigger problems than you.'"

Doris long ago lost the desire to follow current fashions, although she does always try to look nice. To her, that means being neat, clean, and well dressed, with her hair and body groomed. "I don't feel that I am too bad to be as old as I am," she says. "I fix my hair myself because hair means a lot. So many people lose so much of their hair; it's very sad.

"It's sad that some women just give up when they lose their companion. They feel life's over, but it *isn't* if you want to take it," Doris says. "I was so busy doing other things that I never think of sex. At this age there are so many more women than men. The last years of my husband's life, he wasn't well and sex didn't interest me anyway. We cared for one another. It's just up to the individual."

Widowed for 23 years, Doris says she will never marry again. "I've enjoyed myself and dated around because I do like men and enjoy their company," she says. "But they really need someone more than women do: their mamas took care of them, then their wives. I once thought of remarrying but decided I was overage and grayed, and he has since passed away. He would have married if I had wanted to, but I was too selfish. I had my own life to lead and was having fun."

....

Good health and energy gives you more power.

....

Doris likes to visit her friend Elsa, who lives among her peers in an independent-living facility that has four units to a building. "They're all over 72, and some get home care and help from families. I take a covered dish to the clubhouse on Wednesdays... and always find someone I have things in common with," Doris says. "I never felt shunned if I take the trouble to reach out. I like to talk them out of feeling sorry for themselves about age. Especially if they know they're not as old as you are, maybe they can get up and give it a try. Sometimes I need to be firm and tell them: 'Get some backbone and keep moving.' A lot of people don't like to reach out, but I'm gifted and thankful.

"When I was 60 I felt old," Doris recalls, "but once I hit 80, I realized, 'I've got it made.' Now I'm 89 and I run with a bunch of independent women. I don't worry much about growing old. Each of us has a life allotted. If you had goals, you could accomplish what you set out to do. Lots of women wanted to get married and have children. My goal was to be educated and to appreciate everything, which is why I went to college in my fifties."

As body and mind change with the passing years, attitudes change too, Doris observes. "When I meet someone who seems to think, 'I won't pay any attention to her because she's too old,' I try to make a friend of them and tolerate them." Such compassion is a most attractive characteristic of Eighties Women.

. . . .

DORIS FACES FEW IF ANY challenges that she cannot handle in her eighty-ninth year and she shines as an outstanding example of feeling youthful at any age. She remembers feeling old when she was 60 but, 29 years later, she no longer worries about the concept of aging. Now Doris lives each moment as fully as she can, surrounding herself with people she can care about and stay connected to. Even at her advanced age she is taking care of others and spends her time cheering up her peers who are down and out about feeling and being old even though they are younger than she is. Doris still drives and is independent and has spent most of her life taking care of herself. Women who still see their lives as full of opportunity have often spent their lives educating themselves and seeking out the company of like-minded, smart, savvy women who also are independent and self-sufficient. They expect to keep going, driving in high gear to be who-knows-how old. Doris expects to see her one-hundredth birthday, which she says with pride and satisfaction.

The only challenge that might make trouble for a woman like Doris is her reluctance to make plans for the time she is no longer able to care for herself. By putting off making decisions about her home and belongings, she's also avoiding thinking about end-of-life healthcare issues such as naming a durable power of attorney if she becomes unable to speak for herself. Women who are still so healthy and strong find it hard to believe they will ever *not* be able to care for themselves. Even if Doris moves to Elsa's independent-living facility , it does not offer assisted services to the residents. Eventually she or her family will be responsible for hiring additional healthcare aides or they will need to move her to assisted or nursing care if her mobility or health fail her.

Doris offers to her peers an excellent example of a woman who has aged successfully yet still feels youthful and strong. She is connected in her world, she has friends, and she has interests. When women continue to make their days worthwhile and care for others along the way they tend to continue to grow and learn. Eighties women are no strangers to difficult times and they see themselves as more than just survivors: they are thriving and 80-plus years strong. Doris has good psychological health and a strong, vibrant personality and she possesses an intuitive nature to stay connected.

Eighties Women like Doris do not speak easily about their personal issues and are often silent about their own concerns and worries. This may leave them in a potential dilemma when they have to seek outside help. The best way to prepare is to educate themselves about their options during these last years and learn which decisions they can make now. Putting their plans in place will comfort and reassure them and their families as well. Knowing where they can go, what they can afford for the care she needs, and who will act as a personal representative will help women of any age let go of worry about what might happen. So far, Doris has not identified the one person she wants to step in to help her and to see that her wishes are carried out if she cannot voice them herself.

Doris has been a caregiver for others most of her life and she is not used to others helping her. If she does eventually need help, she may find it hard to accept, much less, welcome it with gratitude. It would help for Doris to talk about how she would feel and how she would deal with losing her mobility or her good health. It also is extremely important for her to understand her financial needs and to know that she will not outlive her money. Doris serves as an excellent role model both for women her own age and for those who are any amount younger. She would make a wonderful mentor to any woman.

HELEN: "I DID NOT ANTICIPATE HAVING SUCH POOR HEALTH."

Helen, 86, had always been healthy when she was younger. She exercised and ate sensibly, so her current situation has come as a shock. "I did not anticipate having such poor health," she says. "I feel frustrated by being unable to take a simple walk or unable to clean house for long. I'm even unable to tie my shoes." Although she always thought she wanted to live to one hundred, she has lately abandoned that dream because of her ill health. "I've survived breast cancer, and shoulder and knee surgery. I used to love to travel, but I do not enjoy it anymore because now my back causes me so much pain," she says.

Helen's husband died of a heart attack after 57 years of marriage. "I went in to fix his lunch while he removed a tree house," she recalls. "My neighbor called to ask, 'Is that Frank lying in the back yard?' It took so long for me to quit thinking about it and to get over it. In a way, though, the suddenness was a blessing. My sister-in-law was in a nursing home for two years and used up every bit of their funds."

Losing a spouse wasn't her worst grief. Of her four children, her oldest son died many years ago in a car wreck at age 24. Her only daughter died more recently of a brain tumor, having lived nine years longer than anyone expected. "Her husband divorced her near the end, and she lived with me the last year. Losing my children was one of hardest things I've ever had to do," Helen says. "You have no one to turn to. You just have to make yourself get up and go on. You can do it."

Helen thinks she looks pretty good, considering. She had an eyelid lift last year, but that was more about being able to see than it was about being seen. "More than anything, I want to preserve a sense of dignity," she says. "When I was younger, I was never pretty or beautiful, but I knew how to project a certain glamour. Now, just being attractive and coming across warm and caring is most important to me."

I can't turn back the clock, but I can be the best 86 I can be.

Most women can identify with Helen's wishes for her future. "I don't want to look any older than I am and I'd like to lose another 10 pounds," she says. "Plus, I wish I were healthier, with fewer physical problems and more energy."

Transportation becomes a significant problem for many women in their seventies and eighties because many stop driving and lose walking mobility. This limits their interaction with other people, particularly when they avoid asking for rides. Many of her friends grew fearful and stopped driving, but Helen is determined to continue to drive. "They'd stop for a week or two, then be afraid to start again. That's why I make a point of driving every day, even if it's just around the corner to the grocery, so I don't lose my nerve."

Helen is a pillar of a local group dedicated to increasing voter participation. That's why it particularly annoyed her recently when her opinion was ignored in a political discussion about presidential contenders. "They acted like I wasn't even there!" she says indignantly. "I just want to be respected."

Despite her health problems, Helen continues to do what she can. "I must remain stoic about it," she says. "I like to get dressed up and go out to eat at a festive restaurant because I love good food. That cheers me up and my friends enjoy that too. When I get frustrated, I remind myself 'I can still do this activity, it just takes a little longer.'"

....

I like to tell people that the first 100 years are the hardest — everything after that is wonderful.

....

Helen also values her ability to relate in a positive way and to keep in relationships with others. "I enjoy making people laugh with a small punchline or quip about current goings-on," she says.

Eighties Women like Helen choose to keep very, very active. "I was always very active socially," says Helen, "with friends in theater, my church, my scholarly work, my writing. I'm really busy, and I like having time for all these things that I did not have time for in the past." During times when she is struggling physically, she makes a point of staying in touch by phone and e-mail.

She has seen how a woman's needs change over the course of her life. "At first a young woman wants lots of romance," Helen recalls. "Then she also wants friendship with her husband. Over time, her mate becomes more of an equal, and they enjoy more togetherness. Good friends and companionship become more important, and they become *everything* after you lose your spouse. You've got to stay involved, because when you have no one else to care for, you tend to become selfish."

Helen's beau is barely 80, and at his age, Helen notes, most men are no longer very sexually active. "They want someone to hold them and say nice things and share things together. Sex as we had it when we were young just doesn't exist anymore. So many had surgery for prostate problems. I know from experience," she says with a laugh, "that Viagra doesn't always work. It has a lot to do with circulation and blood flow. The men really miss sex, and I can remember it sure was fun. But we can still be affectionate and give each other a lot as far as caring. Women could probably still enjoy sex, but the man has to be able to perform."

"I suffer from arthritis with terrible pain at times," says Helen. "Sometimes, when I have gotten down on my knees, I can barely get up again. My bad asthma keeps me out of breath and it's getting worse. Will I be able to care for myself in

20 years? I have no idea. I hope I won't be in a nursing home; in fact, I probably won't be here at all because I would be 106 years old!"

Helen did not want to stop teaching college English part time, but her asthma wouldn't allow her to walk in the cold from her car to the building. "I had been busy my whole life, ever since my first job in high school. What bothered me most about retiring — to suddenly quit — is that I felt so unproductive. At first I joined too many clubs and groups but I just couldn't get interested. I was desperate to be busy but I've since learned how to relax."

She worries about her finances. "Did I put enough away? Once you retire your income is pretty much fixed. I do have a pension from the hospital and a broker account but it's not doing too well. I just hope I don't outlive my money," she said. "Still, all the older women I knew when I was younger seemed OK with getting old. But remember, in my generation, women tended to depend on their husbands and now, as then, single women suffer financially."

Helen considers it absolutely vital to strive for goals. "Reaching them is not the most important thing," she believes. "Also, to be a happy old person one must feel needed and wanted, which means you must be more concerned with the lives of others than with yourself." Her advice for women to feel youthful: "Be interested in many areas, be active in cultural groups, have a wide variety of friends. Be understanding of others as much as possible and look for and acknowledge the best in people."

· ·

HELEN'S GREATEST CHALLENGE WILL BE the continuing decline in her health because her options will become increasingly limited. When she stopped driving she had to develop a new definition of her independence. Now, her diminishing lung capacity from chronic asthma is forcing her to curtail many other activities. Although she sees this as a real deficit she is usually able to maintain a positive attitude.

When a woman has to leave a beloved career she may have a hard time finding a good replacement for the stimulation and the satisfaction of gainful employment. That stress adds to worries about declining health and reduced income and she may watch nervously as her living costs creep up. Most women worry that they will outlive their money. These are common challenges for women whose careers did not provide adequate pensions and who have no financial cushion when their lives change.

Helen is a smart woman, which is clearly one of her greatest strengths. She is a good companion and she has stayed connected without isolating herself. Despite her health problems she has found ways to be involved and interested in the world, which helps her feel as youthful as possible considering her physical limitations. Eighties women have plenty of self-reliance to get them through tough times, and they know they need to develop action plans against the day their health no longer allows them to live independently.

When women have done careful financial planning they are able to piece together a safety net with pension, investments, and Social Security income. It's tight, but Helen feels relatively secure, and is grateful to have her supplemental health insurance through her retirement plan. The hardest thing for Helen is going to be finding — and trusting — someone to lean on if she becomes unable to care for herself. When a woman loses a child — and Helen lost two — she feels devastated and may lose her faith that anyone will be there to help her. This is understandable, but women need to work through it. Helen's remaining two children love her and want to help, and have been wondering why she simply will not turn to them. Helen would do well to accept their offers of help and designate one or both of them as her durable power of attorney for health care. By introducing her children to her financial advisors and doctors, an Eighties Woman can feel calmer and more confident that her needs will be met in the way she prefers.

WHAT DO EIGHTIES WOMEN WANT?

Eighties Women are definitely strong survivors. They have lived longer than most of their peers, and their longevity is both a gift and a challenge. Of the women who are 85 or older today, eight out of ten are widows, one in ten is still living with a spouse, and about three in one hundred are divorced.

One of the biggest new challenges that Eighties Women have to face is getting rock-solid with a new self-image that is *not* dependent upon being young, energetic, or beautiful, and that stands up in the face of other people's views, which may be distorted by ageist stereotypes. This self-image must be positive and solid yet also must allow for some release of control and reliance on others.

Maintaining Caring Connections

- ⮑ Keep in touch with friends and family. Do not wait for the call or email or letter. Initiate the contact yourself.
- ⮑ Do not think others are too busy for you. Show love and you will get it back.
- ⮑ Get up each day and fix your face, style your hair, and dress for the occasion
- ⮑ Reach out each day and have a plan for the next day.
- ⮑ Keep your pains and aches to yourself unless you are talking with a professional.
- ⮑ Stay positive. Everyone likes to be around an upbeat person.
- ⮑ Mentor and be a role model for younger women.
- ⮑ Feel good about all you are and what you have to offer to others.
- ⮑ Cultivate a philosophical approach rather than living with anger and regret.

I've heard women say with regret that they wished they had done more to stay young, but it's not as if they could have stopped the clock. True, maybe they could have taken more vitamins or eaten more veggies, but even if they had, they would still be old and need to adjust their view of themselves.

The truth is their enduring value has not lessened as they have become more wrinkled. Quite the contrary. An Eighties Woman is a repository of knowledge, skills, understanding, and support that can help a family through difficult times. As role models for successful aging, they are indeed family treasures.

Nonetheless aging parents and adult children must work out their changing roles. Accustomed to being the caregiver, the Eighties Woman may have to cope with seeing her children start to take control of her finances, her home, her mobility, and even beginning to make decisions about where she lives or what she eats.

These issues can cut to the core of self-esteem. Just because a woman needs her children's help doesn't mean she has stopped being the parent, and her children do not need to "parent" her. That said, children often feel confused and threatened by their changing roles. Some children handle their frustration and distress by getting angry, bullying, or demeaning their aging parents. An occasional flare-up is human nature, but an ongoing pattern of anger and domination qualifies as abuse and should be reported to authorities. Because an older person who feels dependent is unlikely to report abuse, her children, friends, and other family members need to be alert for troubling signs.

In cultures characterized by deep respect for elders, declining abilities do not necessarily bring a loss of status, and an adult daughter would never characterize herself as parenting her mother. Instead, she would take pride in fulfilling her filial duty as part of the natural course of life. She would know that someday her own children would do the same for her. But in a youth-oriented culture, children have not necessarily been taught how to handle this life change with delicacy and respect, and may perceive the parent as taking a childlike role. Eighties Women themselves feel confused, and they ask, "Who am I if I have to ask for help from my children? Can I still see myself as worthy of respect and consideration? Do they still respect me?"

Talking openly with children and other family members can help bring ideas and attitudes out in the open and establish realistic expectations. Eighties Women might think of themselves as advancing into the executive ranks: they must become comfortable with delegating certain tasks while retaining a core sense of self-control and responsibility.

Eighties Women Want Others To Know

- 🖎 I am intelligent. I can still make my own decisions.
- 🖎 I have worked hard and planned carefully to avoid being a burden to my family.
- 🖎 I sometimes am afraid that my body will give out on me and I will not be able to drive and do what I want to do.

EMOTIONS OF EIGHTIES WOMEN

- ❦ Eagerness to make the most of the years ahead
- ❦ Satisfaction with her many accomplishments
- ❦ Fear that her health may fail and leave her unable to care for herself
- ❦ Anxiety about diminishing mental capacity
- ❦ Concern about outliving her money
- ❦ Happiness about being able to say what is on her mind
- ❦ Worries about encountering an unexpected crisis
- ❦ At peace with herself and her spiritual faith
- ❦ Disappointment about getting older despite every effort to prevent it
- ❦ Fear of being a burden to others
- ❦ Delight with her many life experiences

See sidebar next page

EMOTIONS OF EIGHTIES WOMEN

· ·

* Eagerness to share stories with others
* Enjoyment of small moments, free of regret

❧ I worry about losing my partner and about being alone.

❧ I want my children to stop trying to parent me and understand I am still in charge.

❧ I want to feel included and do not want to be dismissed or set aside by the world.

❧ I want to know I have lived a good life and made my mark in this world.

❧ I have much to say and I am tired of worrying about what others think of me.

❧ I love doing what I want to do when I want to do it.

❧ I have faith and comfort in knowing I have done my best.

❧ I want to be respected as a person.

❧ I want others to listen and really hear me.

SO TIRED OF FUNERALS

One downside of great longevity is the pain of outliving spouses, friends, and even children. "I'm getting so tired of going to funerals," the Eighties Women say. Suffering so many losses can leave them subject to depression and isolation, so they have to work extra hard at maintaining good psychological well-being.

Eighties Women who have lived lives full of accomplishment may struggle with facing days and nights alone. Particularly if they have suffered depression earlier in life, they may begin to feel helpless, hopeless, and anxious. This is an ever-growing problem and should be addressed, especially since more and more women will be hitting their eighties and flying onto their nineties and beyond, when by all rights women should be celebrating the richness of their lives. Healthcare systems will need to have professionals available to deal with this growing social problem. When dealing with a broken healthcare system for themselves and spouses, women should talk about their needs with family and friends, bring someone to appointments, and have an advocate attend them any time they must be hospitalized.

Many Eighties Women find themselves energized, however, by the sense that they are running out of time. When they face the fact of very limited years ahead, many excitedly and determinedly plan what to do with their remaining life energy.

Eighties Women Get It Together

If you don't see a good reason below to gather together with other women, make up your own.

- Girlfriend weekend getaways: to the city, country, spa, health club, or movies
- Girls' night out—or in
- Mentor women in your profession or the wider community
- Mall walkers
- Political groups that educate women on the issues and help get out the vote
- Hobby groups: Books, gardening, sewing, knitting, crafting, scrapbooking
- Faith group: Bible study, or study of world religions
- Memory keepers: write memoirs, make books
- Cards or board games
- Philanthropic service groups: create donations for disaster victims (health kits of towel, washcloth, toothpaste, comb, soap); band together to help a friend or church member; support children or victims of domestic violence or the poor.
- Develop a telephone tree for checking on friends who are housebound.
- Share rides to help friends who no longer drive.

ACCEPTING WHAT IS

Every Eighties Woman owes it to herself to become well informed about how to care for herself emotionally and financially. Money is a big issue when women have not earned enough or saved enough to provide comfortably for their old age, or when a health catastrophe decimates their resources. Although it is a behavior especially characteristic of older women, today women of every age still choose to depend on a spouse or some other entity to care for them and their affairs. They cheat themselves by failing to become financially savvy about what the bills are and what it will take to live a long and productive life. Instead of enjoying their golden years, many Eighties Women find they must struggle to make ends meet and worry about their futures and their ability to care for themselves.

NORMAL AGE-RELATED MEMORY LOSS OR DEMENTIA?

Normal age-related memory loss	Dementia
Forgetting names you remember later	Memory gaps that impair daily living
Forgetfulness stays about the same	Forgetfulness gets worse
Forgetting words	Forgetting how to do things you've done many times before
Forgetting the name of a blender	Forgetting how to use a blender
Telling someone a story again	Repeating phrases or stories in the same conversation
Did I pay that bill?	Difficulty handling choices or money
Slower to learn new things	Can't learn new things
What did I come into this room for?	Doing things that require steps, like a recipe
Forgetting which day you did something.	Losing track of what happens each day

Increasing longevity increases the risk of outliving our money. Healthcare costs are rising, and not planning leaves many older women finding their choices limited by government program guidelines or their family's finances. This is an area women need to work to improve — both individually and collectively — because of the increasing numbers of women who are living well beyond their eighties, into their nineties, and even into their hundreds.

Health is, of course, a major concern for most Eighties Women, particularly physical problems that limit mobility and threaten their independence. Having good health care and support is more important than ever, and women need good connections with healthcare professionals and organizations to help them meet their physical challenges.

Although Eighties Women don't like seeing lines and sagging skin in the mirror any more than younger women, they are no longer shocked to see them. By their eighties, most have some level of acceptance of "being old." One thing is certain. We all know how this life ends.

The Plans No One Likes To Think About

- Talk to your family about your plans for the future and how they will be involved.
- Use legal documents to designate your power of attorney and durable power of attorney for health care, and make sure you understand the difference.
- Complete your financial planning, including wills, trusts, executors, or trustees.
- Look realistically at your long-term care plan. If you do not already have long-term care insurance in place, talk with your financial advisor and insurance agent about whether it makes sense for you. Investigate all your options.
- Get clear about end-of-life issues. It's important that you talk openly with everyone who is likely to come to your bedside when you are failing. Be aware that even if you place a Do Not Resuscitate order in your medical record, in reality your healthcare team will follow the wishes of whichever relative demands you get the most care because the doctors will be afraid of being sued.

Looking toward death, even though it may still be 20 or more years off, Eighties Women often find comfort in faith and philosophy. Acceptance may be possible for some women who have faith in a higher power. Whether they anticipate a heavenly life after death when they will be reunited with loved ones, or believe in reincarnation, or have simply arrived at an acceptance that death is the final, natural end to life, women of faith seem to handle old age better than those who are anxious, fearful, and resentful.

NOT TOO OLD TO BE INTERESTING

Eighties Women tell us they have been given this extra time as a precious gift that is too important to waste. They are giving back in whatever ways they can as they seek to make each day stand for something. Eighties Women are most likely to continue to age successfully when they have planned for hobbies and activities they can enjoy as their physical abilities change. It's especially important for

KEEPING YOUR MIND SHARP

············

- 🌺 Exercise and keep physically fit.
- 🌺 Eat a diet rich in antioxidant fruits and vegetables and Omega 3 fatty acids.
- 🌺 Get enough rest.
- 🌺 Read, learn, and grow.
- 🌺 Do routine things in a new and different way: Shower with your eyes shut; drive a new route home.
- 🌺 Surround yourself with interesting people.
- 🌺 Travel to experience new and exciting things.
- 🌺 Do things that challenge you: learn a language, try a new job or skill.
- 🌺 Volunteer and interact with others.
- 🌺 Keep up with current events.
- 🌺 Manage your stress level.

them to continue to learn and grow each day. When they have lots of opportunities for socialization and relationships, they will continue to feel needed and useful and able to reach out to others. When they see their relationships as personal treasures, they love to find someone to listen to the story of their lives. This enables them to share their heritage and pride of family.

Many Eighties Women are benefiting from their lifetimes of wise financial decisions and their families appreciate knowing they have the resources to pay for additional care should they ever need it. Regardless of their income level, it's critically important, since by now most are on fixed incomes, that they have mastered the art of living within their means. Those who have a belief in a higher power and practice their faith on regular basis usually find some comfort. Even those without faith can feel calm if they have personality characteristics that enable them to not spend time worrying or being anxious about their problems. A final key, both for Eighties Women and those at any stage of their lives, is to maintain a positive attitude and to feel in control of at least some part of their lives.

INTO THE NINETIES: SEE YOU AT PILATES!

The statisticians tell us that a woman who celebrates her ninety-first birthday today can expect to live at least five more years to become 96. However, no Nineties Women took part in our original research project, so we won't speculate about their attitudes and concerns in this edition. As part of our ongoing research, we will interview women in their nineties as well as centenarians to learn how women will continue to learn and thrive into their very latest years.

When the Twentieth Century began, a woman's life expectancy was only about 48 years, although a few lived into their nineties and beyond. As a society it is important for us all to find ways to celebrate and acknowledge all those special women who worked to earn our right to vote, to use birth control, to own property, to *expect* to be respected and to live without fear of abuse or violence. Even today, none of these rights is secure without our continuing efforts. As more women live to celebrate their one-hundredth birthday and more, we want them to see their value, their importance, and the gratitude we feel for them.

Dr. Nancy's Kick-Butt Keys for Eighties Women

- Keep moving and exercise in every way possible. Use it or lose it!
- Find ways to maximize mental pleasures as physical energies wane.
- Relish relaxation and contemplation: watch the clouds go by now and then.
- Enjoy every pleasure, whether a great meal, good friends, or good conversation.
- Keep learning and growing each day. You can do both at any age.
- Understand your faith and belief system and share it with others.
- Focus on thanks and appreciation; let go of depression, anxiety, or fear.
- Read, listen to the news, and stay involved so you can talk about current events.
- Stay away from catastrophic (doom and gloom) thinking.
- Stay away from "crystal ball" thinking (you cannot read minds and you cannot predict the future unless you are a certified psychic).
- Stay open to new and exciting things.
- Get out into the beauty of nature at least once each day.

It is time for us all to think about the coming years. If we look around we can all find women who are healthy and vital and strong into their eighties and nineties. Rare? Perhaps, but with luck, our best chance of still being healthy and happy in our later years is to start *now* with consistent good exercise and nutrition, positive mental health, good relationships, and solid financial planning.

We also can see that women coming behind us will have a positive life experience if we work to ensure women are rewarded with equal pay for equal work, are freed from impossible standards of youth and beauty, and will be treated fairly and with respect regardless of their age. When we create this better world, when someone asks: "How old are you?" women will be proud to say their real age, whether they are 20, 40, 60, 80, or 100 or more years old.

Visit www.womenspeak.com to learn more about the eighties. Express yourself and share ways you have learned, grown, and found your best life.

CHAPTER 9   *Women Living, Loving,*
            and Laughing Longer

It's time to move from feeling invisible to being visible.

DR. NANCY

When I began this journey to find out what women really thought about aging in our society ,I knew I had to reach out and listen. Ten years later, the Women-Speak Project applauds the more than 1,200 women of varied backgrounds who courageously spoke out to share their thoughts and emotions, fears and concerns with us. They told us great stories about their personal journeys and what was on their minds. We thank all these wonderful women in their twenties, thirties, forties, fifties, sixties, seventies, and eighties. This book honors all of them.

We have heard from these women in surveys, focus groups, and visits to WomenSpeak.com. They feel unprepared to age successfully; aging is really confusing to them. Aging is like going down a new path in totally uncharted territory. We need to dismiss the myths about this "aging thing." It's a good time for a beauty revolution and revolt to stop women from feeling bad about themselves, whether they are 20 or 50 or 80.

In some cultures the elders are seen as teachers, as the experts in living. The Chinese see age as a sign of maturity and knowledge; they revere their elders, whom they consult, defer to, and respect. Isn't it funny that in the United States we lie about our age as children to appear older and later in our lives we lie to make ourselves younger? Youth and immaturity drive a huge portion of the United States economy. Why? First of all, we are a young country, so what can you expect? But we also have handed our power over to marketing forces that manipulate our fears and dissatisfaction with ourselves to sell us products.

Women are tired of this and ready to demand change. If media and marketers were smart they would realize the opportunity present in supplying women with products and services we really want and need. Won't it be great when women take their 85 percent buying power and demand more from the market, and insist that damaging negative myths and superficial views of older women no longer be tolerated in our society?

We can use our marketing clout to make companies understand that women's priorities are to keep themselves and their families happy and healthy. We need products, services, and information to show us that older women are still visible, that the changes in our bodies such as a loss of muscle are not failures or reasons to feel guilty. As older women we also need encouragement to get our nutrition and exercise plans on track. We want to feel good about our age and feel good about how we look, and we want our daughters and granddaughters to feel the same way. Only when companies support these goals will we become loyal to their brands.

Dove's Pro-Age campaign is a start. At least they are trying to help us feel good about ourselves. Still, women should not feel bad if they don't look as good as the images of Dove's models. According to insiders, those photos were vigorously retouched in Photoshop to remove the true signs of aging.

We believe that women deserve to feel good about themselves no matter their age. We are tired of having to make excuses for ourselves. We want to rejoice in our lives and experiences, and feel free to not only treasure our memories, but to also continue to make new ones.

Women take a stand on aging in so many different ways. Some women join the Red Hat Society and parade around in their purple dresses to show the world they are over fifty and proud of it. But not all women are eager to join the parade. Many emphatically *do not* want to join a women's group, *do not* like getting older, and *do not* want anyone to know their age.

WHAT WOMEN WANT AND NEED

Most experts agree that the best way to stay youthful is to reduce stress. One of the first ways to do this is to have realistic expectations and to stop being so hard on ourselves. Developing healthy ways to nurture our bodies, minds, and spirits will ensure that we can be happy wherever we are.

Women need to know that we make a difference in this world and that with all of our talents we can use our feelings of passion and our purpose and not feel depressed, pissed, or dismissed. We want bliss, lots of bliss. We do not think any woman should feel invisible or excused from life. It is a time for all women to find their voice and come out standing proud and strong.

Your Wonderful Life

Use this checklist to evaluate where you are in your life. Write your answers, focusing on your gratitude for the positive answers and freely expressing your feelings about the negative ones. Note any areas you would like to change, then use this chapter and WomenSpeak.com to help you change the negatives into positives. (Thanks to intuitive Laura Day for the first three ideas which she shared with us on Timeless WomenSpeak Radio.)

- Are you physically and financially safe?
- What do you want? (Not, What do you need?)
- Who do you know who can help you get what you want?
- How do you define success?
- Are you where you want to be?
- Are you healthy, vital, and strong?
- Do your relationships nurture and satisfy you?
- Do you feel in control of your finances?
- Are you afraid of getting older?

What do we have in common? Each of us has reached — or will reach — a point of feeling dissatisfied as we get older. What to do? First of all, women have to dispel the myths and take pride in themselves to change these negative self-images (too fat, too thin, too flat-chested, too old, not pretty, not valued). We want and need to take back our personal power and reinvent ourselves as beautiful women with inner beauty and gifts to share.

WOMEN HELPING THEMSELVES

This chapter focuses on what we can do—and how we can do it—to succeed at feeling youthful and valued at any age. We want to help you find mentors; find resources for your health, your relationships, and your finances; and find ways to help you redefine or, if you choose, to reinvent yourself so you can be all you wish to be.

We want to help, so we are offering you more good ideas on how to better take care of yourself whether you are 21 or 89. Here are some strategies that we hope can help women build better lives and better support systems, and enable them to live fearlessly.

This book is about not giving in or giving up your inner beauty and personal power. What we would really like is for women of all ages to join us and take a different journey, a journey whose destination is a place where we can all feel good about ourselves, inside and out, and be ready to rock and roll.

At any age there is still time to keep it going and for you to keep growing with love, happiness, and joy in your lives. You can stoke that hot, burning passion for living large; you can live out loud with fulfillment and purpose.

We found that women have four major areas of aging concern: their worries associated with growing older in a society that does not value or honor them as older women, their ever-changing relationships, their finances, and their health. These concerns take different priorities at different stages of life, but the things we can do to regain our power at any age have a lot of commonalities.

SELF-IMAGE FEARS

The longer a woman survives, the greater her chance of living a truly long — and ideally healthy — life. Longevity is thought to be largely determined by genetics, but good lifestyle choices, coupled with modern medicine's advanced diagnosis and treatment, have surely added years to women's lives.

We learned that across all age groups, women who are afraid of getting older feel less powerful and less able to change their lives. This shows up in the way they express themselves. Those who were afraid of getting older use passive terms to express their aging concerns, saying they worry about things like "loss of independence, being useless, and the way they will be treated." Fearful women worry their bodies will betray them, and especially that they will lose their mental capacity. In contrast, women who are not afraid of getting older use much more active language. They worry about things that reflect their sense of self-efficacy, such as "not accomplishing all my goals, not being happy with myself, being unable to achieve all I wanted, and succumbing to the will of others." Women who feel some measure of control over their lives are much more likely to feel confident and content with their aging process.

Finding the energy and ability to stay productive and independent becomes an increasingly important issue with each succeeding age cohort we surveyed. Many women also said they really never talked about getting older to anyone and felt like it was some taboo topic. If they were not trying to dye, diet, nip, and tuck to beat the clock they felt excluded from the conversation.

PLASTIC SURGERY: IS IT RIGHT FOR ME?

Increasing numbers of women are choosing to counteract the physical effects of aging with plastic surgery. By no means would we say "Yes" or "No" to any woman who decides to have a cosmetic procedure to change her looks. It's not just Hollywood stars or celebrities anymore. It's your next-door neighbors, your librarian, your child's teacher, your best friend — or maybe even you — who are getting a face lift, some liposuction, or a little laser work done.

Many of these women say they feel better about themselves, their self-esteem improves, and some even say they feel sexier. Now those are all positive things for a woman to experience, right? Her business, right? It's disappointing, however, to listen to women who don't want surgery and hear the way they criticize and condemn the ones who do. Come on, now, women. Considering the messages our society sends out about our appearance, it's a wonder we're not all standing in line for a procedure, so can't you give your sisters a break and not heap your scorn upon them, too?

As a parent, it is troubling when teenaged girls who have not yet had time to grow their own are asking for a boob job for their sixteenth birthdays. We hope their parents would get them some counseling and mentoring to help them develop a stronger sense of themselves before going under the knife. In fact, many plastic surgeons employ a psychologist to help ensure that women have a healthy, realistic expectation of what a procedure will do for them.

Are You a Good Candidate for Cosmetic Surgery?
By Lois W. Stern*

Find out if there are other health issues you should resolve before elective surgery.

- ✐ Do you have a kidney or liver disorder?
- ✐ Do you have a bleeding disorder?

- Are you a heavy smoker or drinker?

- Are you considerably overweight?

- Do you scar easily?

- Do you have any other serious medical condition(s) such as diabetes, high blood pressure, heart or lung disease, or severe allergies?

- Are you currently under treatment or medication for anxiety or depression?

- Do you have a drug problem?

- Are you in the middle of a life crisis, such as divorce or loss of a spouse?

- Have you had many different cosmetic surgery procedures at different times during your life?

- Are you generally unhappy with your overall physical appearance?

- Are you preoccupied or obsessed with a part of your face or body that others do not consider unattractive?

- Are you suffering from depression?

- Are you considering cosmetic surgery primarily as a means to improve your social life, resolve marital conflicts, or please someone else?

If you have answered "yes" to any question above, consult with your physician and/or a mental health specialist before undertaking elective surgery.

* This checklist is excerpted with kind permission from *Sex, Lies and Cosmetic Surgery*, (Lois W. Stern, Infinity, 2006, 2008), www.sexliesandcosmeticsurgery.com.

Know that the person you are inside is what really matters to your life and happiness. If you want to re-paint your walls, go ahead and enjoy the new look. But you and everyone else will know you are still living in the same house.

BODY IMAGE

Many women tell us they grew up with messages that greatly affected their self-images. These messages continue to influence how they see their reflections in the mirror today, and it often does not match up with the way they think it should look. They think they are too fat, too short, too tall, not pretty, or not like other women. We think this way because the images we see on the newsstand or at the grocery checkout counter offer a distorted view of reality. The covers either feature young girls smiling because they are young and beautiful or hideously unflattering pictures of stars hiding from the camera because they look fat and ugly. There are never any pictures of ordinary human females women who look like us and feel fine.

Self-esteem is how a person feels about the inside and the outside. Women who have poor self-esteem have heard messages while growing up that said, "You do not measure up to all the other pretty, thin, smart girls." These messages can have lifelong consequences. Women in our focus groups told us they heard many of these messages and also felt their mothers had a hard time with age and really worried about losing their looks.

Although coping with society's external views of older women can be annoying, women have devised a number of coping strategies. Susan tells her age proudly, knowing that she looks healthy and strong. Marla shrugs it off, ignores it, then vents by laughing and complaining with her friends. Kathy refuses to tell anyone her age because she refuses to be categorized that way. Carol answers questions about her age by replying, "That is only relevant if we're talking about age discrimination." How old are you? If it bothers you to be asked, go ahead and devise a cute remark to deflect what is, after all, a rude question: "Old enough to know better; Young enough to want more; Oh, I'mabout your age; What's it to you?" That way you can leave your age to the imagination of the perceiver.

COUNTERACTING NEGATIVE SELF-STATEMENTS

A fear of aging is not a rational response. It's an emotion. Women who were once embarrassed to tell their age or admit they are past menopause are taking back their personal power. They are coming to understand this aging thing and are refusing to let their age sideline them in this youth-driven society.

First, be aware of — and don't be manipulated by — media messages. Next, identify and face what you are really afraid of. You may want to work with a therapist or a focus group of trusted girlfriends to do this. Is it your appearance? Grim reaper? Poverty? Ill health or pain? Being a burden? Developing a solid sense of your inner value and lasting beauty is a matter of identifying the negative messages you learned growing up and replacing them with positive self-statements.

Negative Message In Your Mind	Replace With a Positive Message
I'm just not pretty.	I have a great smile and eyes.
I look old and decrepit.	I look good for my age.
I am too old.	My knowledge, wisdom, and skills increase daily.
I am helpless.	I make the world a better place.
I am worthless.	I am a valuable human being.
I'm a failure.	I succeed at many things I try.
I hate growing older.	I'm a lucky one to grow older.

Women can learn to find within themselves their own esteem, dignity, and worth. Catch yourself making negative self-statements today and change them to positive ones.

EATING DISORDERS

As we all know, women are susceptible to eating disorders such as anorexia nervosa and bulimia. Body image issues and perfectionism add up to problems for young girls. Women of all ages experience and even die of eating disorders. A woman who has a distorted body image sees her body primarily in terms of some imperfection that she constantly thinks and worries about. Often these women perceive themselves as out of proportion or damaged in some way (nose too big, hips too wide, mouth too small). This condition, along with low self-esteem, can lead to other issues such as eating disorders, depression and anxiety, and other types of phobias. These conditions all warrant medical and psychological intervention with a trained professional knowledgeable in this field of expertise.

It is so important to get the treatment you need as soon as possible. If you or someone you know has an eating disorder (or even if you only suspect it) please get the medical advice and treatment you or she may need. Eating disorders are treatable and a woman can live a full and satisfying life after treatment.

GETTING OVER AGING FEARS

Fear can and often does paralyze a person. We have the emotion of fear for a very good reason: to keep us safe from harm, real or imagined. We can beat our fears by confronting them head on. If you have garden-variety fears like everyone else, such as, "I know I'll fail my math test," "I'm afraid I'll get hurt," and so on, take responsibility for overcoming them. For example, if you are afraid of speaking in public, take a public speaking class or join Toastmasters. Get out there and just do it.

If you do have a serious phobia of driving, going into an elevator, leaving the house, or getting older, don't beat yourself up about not being able to conquer it alone. If you are very afraid of getting older and your fear is making you hate your aging self, get a therapist and start talking to other women. Call your local mental health association for a referral. There are really good therapists out there to help you

There is actually a name for fear of getting older: gerascophobia. But just because it has a name, do not let your fears control your life or your happiness. Do something each day that makes you a little uncomfortable but is new and keeps you fresh and open to possibilities. Many of the very successful women we spoke to said just that: "Do not let fear get in your way." Yes, they had been fearful but had gone ahead and conquered their fears and felt a tremendous satisfaction and reward from doing so.

We were surprised that the Seventies and Eighties Women we spoke with were so interesting and excited about their lives, so here's another tip. Seek out a nice older woman you admire and get acquainted. Ask how she sees her world, and what she thinks of getting older. You may be surprised to find out she is upbeat, positive, and forward-thinking, and this may help remove some of your fears. And read biographies of smart, capable women who came before us. You will be amazed.

IMPROVE YOUR IMAGE WITHOUT PLASTIC SURGERY

- Surround yourself with beauty, artwork, bright colors, good music, healthy foods.
- Get exercise and feel your body move.
- Surround yourself with happy, fun, loving people.
- Get rid of toxic people in your life, the ones who bring you down, belittle you, or criticize you.
- Do not allow anyone to abuse you or neglect you.
- Send out love and people will flock to you.
- Be what you want to be.
- Act "as if" you are beautiful and you *will be* beautiful.
- Your thoughts and actions will make the world a beautiful place to live.

FIGHTING INVISIBILITY

Throughout this book, women of all ages have expressed their concerns regarding their aging process. They have talked candidly about the ways society responds to them as women. Twenties Women feel invisible because they are perceived as being too young. Women in their forties, fifties, and beyond may feel invisible because they are getting older. It is difficult for the women who enter into their mature years — who have lived lives full of experience, knowledge, and talents that they are ready to share and to show the world, who have so much to offer and share with other women in their fields of interest — it is difficult for them to find that their gifts are neither sought out nor appreciated. For these women, fears of aging made them feel like they were disappearing in the eyes of society. Other women, though, have found ways to feel noticed.

Famous actresses have expressed their frustration and dismay at their industry's response to scripts about older people and that feature older actors. The studios ignore such projects. In response, some actresses find their own financial backers and produce, act in, and promote their own movies.

Just as Hollywood actors bump up against stereotypes of aging women, you will too. Don't let it derail your life. Instead, find a way around it. You can produce your own life. Never let anyone or anything stop you from dreaming and creating the life you want. Instead of allowing someone or something else to make you feel invisible, do something about it for yourself. Refire, inspire. Move from *feeling* invisible to *being* visible.

KNOW YOUR MAMAS—LEARNING WOMEN'S HISTORY

Positive role models are important and help young women learn about what is possible. We know our founding forefathers (our papas like George Washington and Abraham Lincoln) but how many young women know their founding foremothers, our mamas like Susan B. Anthony or Eleanor Roosevelt? Women in our history can serve as role models for young women and inspire pride in our women's heritage.

We have forgotten or never knew the important facts about women's vital roles in our history. How many young women realize what it took for women to gain the right to vote in state and national elections? How about women's rights to control their own reproduction or hold a job other than teacher, nurse, or governess; or to hold a job as a married women; or to keep a job while pregnant; or to work in a traditionally male-dominated profession; or to own property, get a loan, develop a business, divorce, and have a voice in any public or legal matter? At the same time that most women know little about these areas of our history, many universities are reducing or eliminating their women's studies programs. What does this mean to all of us? Women of all ages are losing their history and it means many young women will never understand the important role women have played in winning rights for all of us.

It will help women to feel brave and strong if they know their "mamas" pushed their fears aside and took on the really tough issues. What these brave women did was no easy task. Women went to prison for protesting and wanting to have representation in the legal system and to truly live the ideal that "we are all created equal."

It's a shame that society's pressure to maintain their youthful glow distracts women from their desire and ability to crack the glass ceiling that is still high above women of all ages. Regardless of your political beliefs, the progress of more women into higher office is exciting and inspiring. Before she became the speaker of the U.S. House of Representatives, Nancy Pelosi said that one of her hopes was that she could not only break the glass ceiling but would also break the marble ceiling that had traditionally kept women from gaining political leadership roles in our country. Hillary Clinton said it was her dream, and she hoped the dream of women of all ages, to earn and win the most important leadership role of all, namely president of the United States. She came closer than any other woman in history. To continue this progress, women must keep on fighting and talking and planning to develop their future leadership roles.

Learning About Women's History

- ⚮ We need to learn about women's true importance.
- ⚮ Devote one hour each week to learning about women's accomplishments and history.
- ⚮ Use the Internet for research: What women's events happened on this day in history? Which important women were born on your child's birthday?
- ⚮ Use the library to find books and films about women.
- ⚮ Have dinner-table discussions about what you are learning.

QUESTIONS TO HELP IDENTIFY A POTENTIAL MENTOR

. . . .

Have you ever had a mentor before? If yes, was it another woman or a man? How did the relationship develop?

❀ If you have not had a mentor, think back to when you first knew what you wanted to be "when you grew up." Who and what helped you make your decision?

❀ Who has helped you achieve your current position as a leader in the community and in your field?

❀ How have role models helped shape your leadership style and roles? Where did you find these role models?

❀ What are you willing and able to offer to other women who are entering or advancing in your field?

see sidebar next page

🐚 Take a trip to a place of local or national importance to women—plan by what you are learning.

🐚 Take your children to vote—tell them when and how women won the right to vote.

🐚 Tell your own family stories of struggle and opportunity, for instance, How Grandma got her first job as a weathergirl; When Great-grandma was fired because she got married; How Great-Aunt Sue kept the economy going during World War II; the story of the first woman astronaut.

ROLE MODELS AND MENTORS

People usually believe and behave as they were taught, and women who had poor role models for aging often worried about aging, just like their mothers did. Women who had positive role models more often saw the strength, wisdom, and importance of age and its rewards. Women and girls need positive role models in order to develop realistic views of their bodies and positive self-esteem.

We are so hard on ourselves and on other women. Do you judge yourself harshly? Do you criticize or condemn other women for the way they look, act, dress, talk, and laugh? Please stop! Instead of judging and condemning, try mentoring someone. That is the only way women will retain and regain their personal power, whether they decide to go into business for themselves or choose to leave the workplace to rear children.

Many young women say they are sad and disheartened by the absence of older women role models who are willing to mentor them. Too often women, especially in the business world, seem determined to obstruct other women rather than give them a helping hand. Maysie, 27, says, "The senior women in my office smile and say they want to support me but when I really need their help, I get the cold shoulder. I try to help the new girl and help her with all the office politics and show her the ropes."

That said, younger women might not always have a realistic view of the sacrifices required to advance in a corporate world. Older women express annoyance at young gals who expect opportunities and rewards to come without cost. Younger women need to accord older women their due: respect and support.

The key to women helping women of all ages to successfully live, love, and laugh longer is mentoring. Start today to be or find a good mentor.

One of the best things we can do for ourselves is to open up to other women to give and receive support. Prioritizing time with women friends pays off with fun and it reduces anxiety and depression. Choose a strategy in these pages for building a women's network. Start a Timeless Women group, or a movie or book club. Find a walking partner, join an existing organization, find a mentor in the workplace, become a mentor in the community, and volunteer. Women who are just not that social could try journaling, meditation, spiritual practice, counseling, or psychotherapy.

Experts say it takes 27 days to establish a new habit and we all know how easy it is to bail out before the habit is set, especially with things that frighten us. Joining with a friend or mentor can hold us accountable and keep us working toward our goals. Mentors can show us how other people

QUESTIONS TO HELP IDENTIFY A POTENTIAL MENTOR

* What would have helped you early in your journey down your path of interest?

* What lessons have you learned that might help women who are considering entering your profession?

* What are some pros and cons of women's position in your field today? Has the situation changed in the last 10 years? If so, how and why?

* Would you consider becoming a mentor to another woman?

deal with similar problems and that there are many ways to gain needed knowledge and resources. They can help us believe in ourselves by reassuring us we are not crazy.

A mentor is a person who is successful, admirable, and who has arrived at places her mentoree wishes to go. A woman usually wants to be like her mentor in some ways — perhaps she is a good teacher, communicator, cheerleader, support, or role model. Ethics and honesty are important, but don't expect her to be perfect. A woman also may learn what she doesn't want from a mentor.

To approach someone about becoming a mentor, a woman should look around in her community. Is there someone she admires for her skills or success? Someone she could invite for coffee, or on a walk, or just telephone to ask for advice. She might say, "I admire you and would like to learn from you." She might ask, "What advice do you have for someone like me?" Everyone is pleased to feel admired, and remember — women are happy to help. Once she opens up to the relationship, a woman will identify ways she can help her mentor in return, or at least show her appreciation and pass it on by helping others.

Not every one is suited to be a mentor. What if she refuses? Realize she may already be too busy and overloaded with protégés to take on another. In that case, a woman can tap into her own inner wisdom by pretending to have a conversation in which she asks for advice. Acting "as if" she is talking with her wished-for mentor gives her a chance to practice thinking outside of her usual perspective. She can also buy an author's book and learn from her written words.

The relationship should feature good rapport and it helps (but is not essential) for them to like each other and have similar learning and working styles. Women have mentors they talk with by phone, e-mail, or face to face; sometimes weekly or monthly, sometimes much more rarely. There is no perfect schedule, especially because mentors are often very busy individuals. Most successful women have more than one mentor to turn to in different times and situations.

As in any relationship there are potential pitfalls. Levels of dependency or confusion can develop, and it's important to be clear about why the person is willing to become a mentor, particularly to avoid uncomfortable hidden agendas. Note: A mentor is not necessarily a woman's banker, therapist, chauffeur, babysitter, secretary, lover, or confessor.

A mentor is only one of the many variables a woman needs, and no one person will have all of the answers. A woman needs to continue to broaden her scope of resources when she enters any new area of interest. Growing and expanding her horizons will ensure that a woman stays up to date and marketable.

CHANGING OUR OWN LIVES

A baby girl born today will have an 80 percent chance (it gets better each year) of reaching her hundredth birthday. More and more women are already reaching their hundredth birthday and tell us how they did it. Some say they ate well and exercised, some drank nothing or some drank a martini or two, many just had fun, some prayed, some exercised and pumped iron, and most were surprised they made it.

Regardless of our final number of days, each of us has an opportunity to re-invent ourselves many times. Many women are doing just that and say it is one of the very best things about getting older. Once they reach maturity and have had the job, raised the family, and made the money, they take time for themselves. Our older years present us with a fantastic opportunity to say: "At last, time for me." They told us stories of what they had to do and then what they had dreamed of doing. Often we heard women talking about what was in their hearts and what passions flowed in them and the desires they had. We found many women want to make a difference in this world and to leave some sign that they existed. They wanted to give back and they felt the call to find their purpose and passion and create something amazing.

For the first time they were not apologizing any longer but putting themselves first. They were finding a personal trainer to help get their bodies strong and sexy. They were working out in a women-only gym to focus on building strength and confidence for themselves alone. They were getting their "sexy back," or happily turning their backs on sex; either way, they loved their lives and the way they felt. They were contracting with life coaches to begin their journey of self-examination to find self-fulfillment and personal satisfaction. They were joining with other women for encouragement, support, and inspiration. In so many ways they were discovering or taking back their personal power.

Women also were taking into account that giving back to other women was key to their own personal development and efficacy. By mentoring other women they could share their gifts and dreams. Self-esteem rose in all of the women who felt they had achieved self-actualization and their true selves. We can learn much from them.

Women hunger for other women to help them and to role model for them. Women in the media like Oprah Winfrey, in entertainment like Celine Dion, in film like Goldie Hawn, in politics like Hillary Clinton or Condoleezza Rice, can inspire women to celebrate each other. We can do so much to help ourselves and raise each other's self-esteem and this is essential for all women and girls if we are to grow as strong, smart, independent women. Women are strongest when they develop their own "locus of control" within themselves to change their worlds.

LAWS OF ATTRACTION

The ancient laws of attraction have taught us to visualize what we want "as if" it is what we already have. We are what we think we are. Women are powerful creatures and have the ability to create their own reality moment to moment. Why is one woman happier and more satisfied with herself and her body than another woman? It's pretty simple. The woman who is happy with herself has lots of positive self-statements stored in her brain. She wakes each morning feeling she can make her day and create her world to her benefit. She sees herself as able to make good choices that will have positive outcomes. If she chooses poorly she also takes responsibility for the consequences. Women who use these strategies are successful in life, love, and aging.

Any woman can easily develop these strategies and with practice find herself living more fully and with passion and fulfillment. We get what we put out there. Yes, we all have heard of The Secret and the ancient laws of attraction.

It's not brain surgery. We get what we ask for and if we keep our eyes open we will notice that what "stuff" we put in our brains has a really good chance of showing up on our doorsteps. We often hear from women who ask "Why do I keep finding myself in the same dead-end job, or the same crappy relationship, or feeling so bad about myself?" We ask these women to consider, "Why do you keep choosing the same thing over and over again?"

Put out into the universe what it is you want. We feel confident you will get what you are asking for. Be careful and be cognizant to ask for the positive things and also make sure you feel you are deserving of goodness and positive things. Be clear what your self-statements are each day. Do not innoculate yourself with negatives of any kind. Believe your life can be good and you will receive goodness.

RELATIONSHIPS: HEAVEN OR HELL?

From mates to parents to children to co-workers, it's our relationships with other people that make our lives worthwhile—or a living hell. It is hard to imagine how many women today are suffering and living with abuse and violence. Each of us needs to do what we can to stop domestic violence in our society; it's not OK. Too many men still tell their women, "Shut up and do what you're told." Invite a woman to do something and far too often she will still say, "I'll have to ask my husband if it's OK." How many of us are still allowing someone or something to block our success, our well-being, and positive self-esteem?

Caregiving for others is an important role for most women, whether for our children, our parents, or our friends. Women everywhere struggle with balancing their traditional roles at home and in the community with their new opportunities and responsibilities in the workplace. Unfortunately, young mothers often feel criticized, whether they work outside the home (guilty for neglecting their families) or not (guilty for not bringing in income.) Society is no easier on women who compromise by working part time.

When my ob/gyn attends the weekly staff meetings at the hospital the topic often turns to units of service (number of patients seen per day) and overall productivity results for each clinic and hospital. She says. "My goal is not to be the most productive, busy doc on the block. I do want people to understand that I am a working mother who also wants to have a good family life. I do not want to be one of the boys and work 60-hour weeks and spend all my time away from my family. I often feel I am perceived as being less dedicated and interested in my career since I don't want to sacrifice my home life to my medical career."

What surprised her most is the way her female colleagues seem to expect that motherhood and family life must of course come second if one is to have a successful medical practice. Until businesses — and women themselves — can formulate and accept standards that enable them to fulfill their goals as wives, mothers *and* workers, women will continue to feel conflicted about their multiple jobs. Women today have a unique opportunity to create for themselves the comfortable employment opportunities they crave.

CREATING THE RELATIONSHIPS YOU WANT

Developing lasting relationships and understanding your personal needs are crucial for successful aging. Learning to ask for what you want in every relationship — whether with spouse, children, friends, or associates — certainly increases the likelihood that you will get it. If you don't feel you can ask for what you want, it's time to find out why, and make some changes.

Why not take responsibility for yourself and let others do the same? When members of the sandwich generation take on increasing responsibilities for aging parents as well as their children, something has to give.

Another important area for planning is your late-life living arrangements. It's highly likely that long-lived women will need some assistance in their final weeks or years. Depending on your circumstances, long-term care insurance, multistage retirement communities, a mother-in-law apartment in an adult child's home, and savings for home care might all be part of the mix. A variety of intentional communities are springing up around the country. These include co-housing, an idea imported from Denmark, in which people — including single women — live in their own homes while sharing a commons building with cooking, laundry, and social facilities. Many such communities are developing nationally, each with an individual flair.

Women who begin talking and planning early can have the satisfaction of making their own decisions right up to their last days. Their families, especially their children, are so grateful.

Improving Your Relationships

- Develop a good relationship with yourself. If you do not like yourself who in the world will?
- Get some reality therapy: Am I crazy? Do I deserve more?
- Practice the laws of attraction. What you send out returns to you multiplied.
- Work out and get fit and ready for anything that comes your way.
- Make a list of what you want out of your relationships with men and women.
- Expect the best and do not settle for less.
- Spend time with people who are fun, make you feel good, and lift your spirits.

- Join clubs such a biking, hiking club, or a Stitch and Bitch" group.
- Get out and about: Travel and see what is out there.
- Try an online dating service with a good reputation.
- Be fearless in life and love.
- If you are unhappy, do something about it.

FAITH

A little over half of the women we surveyed reported they had a church affili-ation, and most of those women said their faith helped in their everyday lives. There's an important connection between having faith in a higher power that helps women cope with all types of life issues. Having faith in a higher power helps a woman to sort through all the messages she hears each day to find spiri-tual peace and tranquility. We all need a helping hand some days, and whether we find it in an organized church, yoga class, meditation, or just private prayer, it can help a woman a lot. This basic coping strategy can help in everyday living and in times of crisis. Having faith and being prayed for may even help people heal faster. Miracles *do* happen. We believe there are many paths up the mountain and whichever path you take is a benefit to you and those you love.

MONEY TO LAST A LIFETIME

Princess is a word most little girls learn around age two and by three years old they have it down to a fine science. They can spell the word and can tell you every story they have ever heard (and there are lots of them). Ask a little girl what a princess does, and the little girls will quickly say they wear beautiful gowns and sparkling tiaras. Ask if princesses do anything in addition to looking beautiful and the children will look at you in amazement: Of course not!

Most of these little cuties also will tell you they want to be or are a princess and they will in fact find their prince one fine day. Many women, especially but not exclusively older women, have cast their husbands in the role of a Prince Charm-ing who takes care of everything for them. These women often felt ill prepared to manage their financial affairs when death or divorce ends their marriages.

Why do we do this to ourselves? Did you ever hear in school "'girls are not good at math"? Don't you believe it. I did until I had to take three classes in research and design to get my doctorate and discovered I could do just fine. Women are still among the poorest in our nation and single mothers may struggle just to keep food on the table. Divorce, illness, and death are leaving many women with their underwear hanging out. Time to start taking business classes and teaching our daughters early how they can support themselves well. Women are living longer by themselves than ever before, so financial security is crucial for a reasonable old age. Remember: *Prince Charming Isn't Coming,* as author Barbara Stanny says in her book by that title, in which she explains how women can gain control of their finances. She also notes that women must *expect* to be wealthy and self-sufficient if they are to achieve those goals.

MONEY MANAGEMENT

If your dollars don't seem to stretch as far as your years, plan to work as long as you can at the highest salary you can. You'll get higher Social Security benefits and have fewer years to fund in retirement. Three-fifths of retirees plan to work at least part time to preserve their spending power.

Improving Your Finances

- Get good financial advice today.

- Invest and save now and do not wait. If you have *no* money left over to invest, examine your income and budget. Get serious about finding ways to spend less and earn more.

- Sign up for any plans at work, profit sharing, 401k; think long-term investing.

- Attend financial planning seminars regularly.

- If you are in debt, get out of debt immediately. Pay off credit cards first. Call local consumer credit counseling organizations in your community for help.

- Learn to advocate for yourself. Most retailers you buy from are looking for permanent customers. You can be one and ask for discounts when you feel appropriate.

- Join a Money Club (WIFE.org) or investment group and ask other women to help you.

- Sometimes it's hard to see the leaks in our budgets. Likewise, we may not be able to see that we are not in fact trapped in that dead-end job. Seek out the truth.

- Trade childcare or services with friends and invest the savings.

JOBS/CAREERS

Many twenty-something women said that they had not hit their head on the glass ceiling but some of the older women (professors) in their forties or fifties sometimes reported that the glass ceiling did exist, but again, they were not hitting their heads but were being held down by the Velvet Anchor. I was told indirectly that women entering the field of psychology "were going to ruin the profession." What is interesting about the results of the surveys is that the younger women felt they had "made it" and yet they had not launched themselves into the workforce to the degree that the older women had. The older women were the ones who expressed having difficulty with job selection and job advancement. Many of the older women were now feeling the weight and struggle to compete and get ahead of their male counterparts. Women's satisfaction level in the workplace also was dependent upon whether they had a mentor and someone who would show them the ropes. Women of all ages felt that women were not good at mentoring and oftentimes felt they were in direct competition with any and all women they worked for or with. Women who had been lucky to find a female mentor in or outside the workplace seem to find a safe harbor and healthy ways to advance and to grow in their jobs.

BEATING THE COMPETITION

Because women have been taught their looks are the most important thing about them, many fear they will no longer be able to compete if they lose their looks. We also have heard from women that covert competition between mothers and daughters causes some girls to get the message that they should not get too pretty or too smart. Women are trained covertly to devalue their capabilities (smart, talented, strong, competent, capable, and assertive) and instead learn to manipulate others into meeting their goals.

We have found that many women are not supportive of one another and basically are not very nice to each other. Women do not seem to rejoice in another women's success and often resent and criticize one another. Only we can change that and only we can be our own champions. We must not succumb to these pressures and allow the covert actions and attitudes of women to keep us all down and feeling bad. Women need to compete with one another in a healthy and open fashion. It has taken me some time to understand that women have this power and we need to stop blaming men and stop making excuses. Who or what is keeping us down? Women can change this and stop feeling defeated or defensive about our lives.

It is OK for us to compete, but keep it above the belt. Men can smile and say to another man, "I am going to beat you." If a woman says that, she is immediately labeled a bitch, plainly *not nice*. Women can help themselves by being more upfront about healthy competition and quit hiding the simple truth: they want to compete and that it is healthy process if done fairly and openly.

COPING WITH COMPETITION

Competition is a healthy form of behavior. Taking part in athletics and working in teams or organized groups are good ways for young women to learn to work effectively and compete in healthy ways with one another.

The world works — and business works well — with healthy competition. Women in business and industry can mentor and teach younger women how to perform and work in these arenas. Healthy competition can help women feel accomplished and valued for a job well done; it builds positive self-esteem and self-images. Mothers need to learn and teach their daughters about healthy competitive skills. This is a life skill women need if they are to be independent and competent in whatever life path they wish to take.

That said, one of the greatest gifts women can bring to their families, communities, and businesses is the understanding that cooperation is often a better model for progress. Competition creates losers as well as winners, while cooperation seeks the good of all. Although it's good to learn how to be a good loser, it is not necessary to view life as a win/lose proposition. Seeking common ground for mutual benefit comes naturally to many women, and these abilities are transforming many workplaces for the good. Women can truly benefit by using their excellent communication skills to bring all parties to the table where they can resolve, plan, and create positive outcomes.

GET A BETTER JOB

Many women feel OK about their jobs and their status in the job market, even though many come out short on the pay scale and retirement funds. Part of the shortfall results from taking time off to care for family, but a lot of it, statisticians say, is just caused by the fact that employers pay women less in many fields.

Most women have worked outside the home at some time in their lives. However, even those who work full time earn much less than men working in comparable jobs. For example, in one Midwestern community (population 325,000) women working full time in professional occupations earned 54 percent of men's wages, according to a recent census. Naturally, this means that women also get smaller pensions, if any, and smaller Social Security checks. These financial realities make aging a penny-pinching prospect for most women.

Around twelve percent of women over 65 live below the poverty level, meaning their income is less than $9,000 per year. The rate for Hispanic and African American women is nearly twice that. The answer is education and training to acquire better job skills.

If you are thinking, "Gosh, I'd be 65 (or whatever) by the time I graduate in four years," think of this: In four years you'll be 65 anyway, just without the extra qualifications to make your last earning years the most profitable ever. You have taken the trouble to read this — you have the skills necessary to improve your lot in life. Get busy.

Everyone feels frightened and insecure about things they do not understand. Take charge of your finances and find someone you trust who will not talk down to you. Never just sign and mail anything someone else gives you. Make sure you *understand* your Social Security benefits, your tax returns, and your investments. Keep asking questions until you do. Take classes, attend seminars, do what it takes to learn what you need. Be fearless. Do things that make you uncomfortable so you will stay ready and

ARE YOU REALLY TRAPPED?

When it comes to your job, if you do not think and act "as if" you were a valuable employee, who else will think you are?

- Ask for feedback on your skills.
- Ask what you need to do to excel.
- Find support for acquiring new skills; make yourself more valuable.
- Learn to sell yourself. Practice your pitch to your boss (why I deserve a raise or promotion).
- Find a female mentor who is successful in the field you are in or wish to enter.
- Start a business venture with another woman.
- Network to find a higher-paying job.
- Look at retirement plans and sacrifice current salary for good benefits.

open to change and opportunity. Keep your options open and your eyes open to possibilities.

CAREER/RETIREMENT/REFIREMENT

Retirement is passé. *Refirement* and renewal is nouveau. After 20 or 30 or more years in one job, you may want something different. Why not figure out a variation on going back to school? You could finish a degree, pursue a second or advanced degree, take a continuing education course or vocational training, attain a certificate or license, attend an online course, or take an evening class. Scrutinize all the schools within your possible distance and prioritize those with services and assistance for adult learners. Investigate all your financing options with a qualified financial advisor.

Talk with counselors about creative ways to meet — or waive — the admissions requirements. Life experience can count for a lot. If you start to feel freaked out about being an older student, use in-school counselors and support to relieve anxiety. Best of all, you can start slowly and ease up to a fuller schedule.

A note about passion and purpose: Our communities would shrivel up and die without the intelligent and devoted volunteer service of women. What would we do without the services of the Red Cross, the United Way, or our local Ys? However, the term *not-for-profit* is outdated. It's a negative way to refer to the organizations whose value systems include so much more than monetary gain. We prefer the term *social profit*. All of our social-profit organizations make our communities better places to live.

We also believe that women should get paid for their work if they need the money. Find your passion and purpose and you may find a new career. If you love to bake, then bake to sell. It really can be true that if you do what you love, the money will follow.

Ask yourself: "What am I passionate about? How do I want to spend my time? Who do I want to spend time with? How do I want to make a lasting mark? What do I want to pass on to others?"

Brainstorm different ways your skills could be put to use, then test-drive it: volunteer, take a part-time position or internship, or take a leave of absence to try it out for a while. You may find you can balance time and money in new ways. For example, many social-profit agencies might offer time off rather than higher salary.

STAYING HEALTHY

Although many women mentioned a generic concern for "health," in our surveys, very few mentioned specific conditions and nearly all seemed unaware of their true risk of various diseases. In reality, women face a host of health problems, including AIDS, osteoporosis, Alzheimer's, urinary incontinence, obesity, arthritis, and mental illnesses including major depression, anxiety, and phobias.

We know women are caregivers and take great pride in caring for others' health needs. Their families typically benefit from their actions but what is discouraging is that women spend more time taking care of others than themselves. In general, women perceive themselves as healthy, but many studies, including ours, show they are in denial about their true health risks. As a president of the National Council on Aging stated, "If women don't get the right information about their risk for disease, they may make wrong decisions about their health."

This blind spot can be life threatening. One out of two women's deaths each year is caused by heart disease; in comparison, just one woman in 30 dies of breast cancer. More than one-third of women who have a heart attack will die within one year, and two-thirds of women never fully recover. Nearly half of women who suffer a heart attack become disabled with heart failure within six years.

Heart disease is diagnosed at a later stage in women and is treated less aggressively. Women aged 65 and older are more than twice as likely to die of heart disease than to die of cancer, and much more likely than men to die within a year of a heart attack (38 percent vs. 25 percent). More women than men die of heart disease each year, yet women still make up only 25 percent of participants in heart research studies.

A woman's best chance to survive a heart attack is to not have a heart attack. She must do whatever she can to prevent heart disease and stroke. One of the most important steps she can take is by controlling her levels of stress and taking care of herself.

Women's Heart Attack Symptoms

Women experience different warning signs of heart attack than men, which may be why women wait longer before seeking help.

The most common early warning signs women experience in the weeks *before* a heart attack are not chest pain but:

- Unusual fatigue
- Sleep disturbance
- Breathlessness
- Anxiety
- Racing heart
- Arms feel heavy or weak

During a heart attack women report:

- Shortness of breath
- Weakness
- Unusual tiredness
- Cold sweat
- Dizziness
- Nausea
- Arms heavy or weak

Women often believe they have gall bladder trouble rather than heart disease. We also are more likely than men to die or become disabled from heart disease. Learn a woman's warning signs of heart attack and pay attention to messages from your body.

Half the causes of the top killers of women are linked to behaviors that we can change. Together, heart and blood vessel diseases (including stroke) kill 34 percent of women in the United States. All types of cancer combined cause 22 percent of women's deaths. Yet, 61 percent of women in one study said they were afraid of cancer, and only 9 percent mentioned heart disease. One of the most important decisions women can make is to get checkups to catch potential problems early and especially to practice a healthy lifestyle.

We did hear many older women felt that their healthcare system had let them down. They told us they felt dismissed and invisible especially after they entered menopause and their childbearing days were over. This is a bad combination. Here we had women denying their own health risks, yet those who asked for the attention of their healthcare providers were made to feel their complaints were all in their heads.

In fact, women are more likely than men to be diagnosed with mental health issues like depression and anxiety disorders, and our hormones can play a role.

"If women have suffered depression in the past, especially if it is postpartum depression or severe PMS, these women may have more depression during the perimenopause when the hormones are wildly fluctuating," says WomenSpeak's health expert Dr. Deb Hill-Busselle. "Once a woman is menopausal, giving them estrogen does not make them less depressed, nor is there an increase in depression due to lack of estrogen in the menopause. However, during the perimenopause, estrogen *can* help reduce depression in women who have had depression in the past and it has now become worse."

Dr. Deb went on to point out that a lot of women's depression is due to life changes: midlife crisis, empty nest, elderly sick parents, financial worries, realizing you married a jerk and have wasted 30 years (joke). "Unfortunately, when women could benefit from a great counselor or even antidepressants, they often just get labeled menopausal, when they really are depressed," she concludes. It is critically important for women to understand their risks and insist that their doctors take them seriously.

MANAGING STRESS

Women are born worriers. If you get tired of worrying ask another women to step in for you while you either crash and burn or just take a mental moment out of the race.

Women are superb multitaskers, able to keep the people, places, and things in their lives running well and on schedule. Women also are born caretakers, and many will not allow themselves to even consider their own needs until they have taken care of *everyone* on their lists. In fact, some women feel guilty at the thought of taking any time at all for themselves. This positions women to obsess about the minute details of other people's lives while completely ignoring their own huge unmet needs.

Unfortunately, this means many women walk around in a permanent state of stress. The *stress response* is important for the survival of the human race. It is a reaction of the autonomic nervous system that helps a woman adapt and respond to the world's many pressures. The autonomic nervous system controls key organs that respond in time of crisis or danger. The stress response prepares the heart, lungs, and muscles to respond quickly to whatever emergency or crisis occurs. Under normal circumstances the body remains calm and balanced. When stress occurs the body gears up to handle the incoming danger.

What happens if a person worries constantly? If stress levels stay high, a woman becomes susceptible to disease or other health issues. For example, severe headaches, digestive upset, depression, anxiety, ulcer, colitis, high blood pressure, skin diseases, muscle pains, irritable bowel syndrome, or even worse, a full-blown heart attack or stroke can all be symptoms of excessive stress. A woman who worries a lot and spends much of her day trying to balance the worlds of others while ignoring herself will sooner or later develop health problems. The take-away message here is a woman needs to learn to manage her stress response to restore balance in her own mind, body, and spirit.

Fortunately, women are beginning to understand that they *can* change the way they feel. They are realizing that if they continue to deny their feelings, nothing will change. But women *can* change their reality by sharing and learning from one another. It's as simple as that.

GET OUT FROM UNDER BEING OVERWHELMED

Women should consider getting outside help and resources for their busy lives. We have heard so many women tell us "I should be able to do this by myself, so I must be inadequate." Who says? Women need to stop being so hard on themselves, accept some help, get over their guilt, and take a first-class seat instead of sitting at the back of the bus.

Learn to say No to others and Yes to yourself. And be as good a friend to yourself as you are to others. Would you demand from a friend what you ask of yourself? Start learning to say No to simple requests and build from there. With practice it gets easier and it may save your life while you teach someone else an important life lesson in responsibility.

GET A CHECK-UP

Migraine headaches are no laughing matter. "One in four women between ages 18 and 49 years have migraines, yet less than half of them have been diagnosed," says Dr. Deb. "There is such a hormonal connection, and there are certain hormonal manipulations that can done to reduce migraines."

Another reason that women need a check-up, Dr. Deb says, is that genetic testing can now determine who is at risk for hereditary breast and ovarian cancer as well as endometrial, ovarian, and colon cancer. In all of these hereditary cancers, women get it early and there are usually multiple family members who are affected. Knowing if you have the gene can drastically change your medical management and empower you to have increased medical surveillance, risk-reducing surgery, and even take medications to decrease the risk."

This chapter includes brief, straightforward information about women's health risks, things they can do, and inspiration from other women who have decided to take control of their own health. Simply by changing their mindsets, including their self-talk, they can build better health and reduce their risk. Women need to learn and understand that it is all well and good to be a caregiver but they also must be sure to look after their own health needs. We must remember we are very different from men and may need different treatments. Find a doctor who specializes in women's health to ensure you get the necessary examinations and treatments.

Talk with your doctor to evaluate your risks for your age and family history. Have regular exams for all body systems, eyes, ears, body, and female issues including breast cancer screening and Pap tests. Ask about how often you should have a stress test to determine your cardiovascular system health and in-depth screenings for bone deterioration.

If you are at high risk for breast cancer, you may need to start having mammograms much younger than 40. Women are being diagnosed earlier and earlier with breast cancer and are surviving because of early diagnosis and treatment. Have your dermatologist check out any changes in moles, warts, and other discolorations in your skin. Hormonal changes can be a real health issue for women going through perimenopause and menopause. Find and talk with a knowledgeable doctor about your symptoms. You do not have to suffer in silence. Ask about the screening tests for ovarian and other gynecological cancers, and make sure your doctor feels your ovaries during your next pelvic exam.

Women must demand good health care. Even more important, they must learn to advocate for themselves and other women. Change will occur only when we take a stand and insist that we receive fair and equal health care.

FOCUSING ON SELF-CARE

Achieving good health for women is a circular process of making sure all systems are in balance. This is called homeostasis and simply means that body, mind, and spirit are all in balance and working cooperatively to create good health. This requires that women do things for *themselves* that make them feel good. Don't be a martyr. A woman should assume a management role; by changing her mindset she can behave "as if" she were the "CEO of herself."

When you confront a serious health issue in yourself or a family member, prayer circles or support groups can help sustain you and offer lots of good coping skills. Check with your local support organizations, like the American Heart Association, the Alzheimer's Association, and many others that offer education, advocacy, and support groups.

Recognize your health risks and identify why you have been in denial. Get information to reduce your risks and become an advocate for yourself and for other women who do not have access to affordable health care. You can set an example. Start today to develop a healthy lifestyle for yourself and teach your children now about good health.

We must break this disgraceful cycle of women and children growing up in one of the richest nations in the world, yet experiencing hunger, poverty, and ill health. By starting early to teach wellness in schools we can help children care for one another. Teaching a child to be responsible for her health starts at birth with regular check-ups and examinations, inoculations, life-skills training, exercise, and regular physical activity. Children also need to learn about giving and helping others to develop healthy self-images and self-esteem. We must help all of our children learn to respect themselves and others.

EXERCISE FOR FUN

Women need to combine weight training, core work, and aerobics into their daily routines. We know that much disease can be kept at bay with exercise and a strong immune system. This system, if kept healthy, can keep heart disease, stroke, breast cancer, diabetes, and other health concerns away. Exercise is the apple that keeps the doctor away. Take a bite and keep moving. After menopause a woman will replace one pound of muscle with fat each year unless she exercises to maintain muscle mass.

Find out what you like to do for exercise and build it into your lifestyle. Get professional guidance about what is right for your age and condition. Learn proper stretching techniques to remain agile and flexible. Much pain and loss of mobility could be eliminated by adequately stretching muscles and tendons.

EATING PATTERNS

Stop dieting. Stop starving yourself. Diets don't work, period. That doesn't mean it is not important to maintain a healthy weight. In fact, the dietary programs for preventing cancer, diabetes, heart, and blood vessel diseases all require attaining and maintaining a healthy weight.

The secret is to learn to eat for life by mastering the basics. Probably most important in this age of obesity is simple portion control. *Stop eating when your hunger is satisfied* and in time your weight will return to normal. When you learn to eat well, you will relish and delight in fruits and veggies, eat low-fat foods and complex carbohydrates, and reduce and/or eliminate sugars and caffeine. Educate yourself about nutritional supplements (like fish oils and vitamins A, Bs, E, C, D) that might help you achieve and maintain better health. Alcohol is full of empty calories. Although more men than women use alcohol heavily, women seem to be more susceptible to diseases associated with heavy alcohol use. Make a plan for eating right when you go out. Many restaurants offer healthy choices so ask your server about healthier options or have half your meal boxed to take home. It turns out that a few simple remedies, lifestyle changes, and commonsense approaches can do a lot to extend your life.

BECOMING VISIBLE

What women need isn't a makeover to change their looks, says former *Ladies Home Journal* editor and author Myrna Blyth. Instead, they need to change the way they feel inside about the way they

BUILDING A HEALTHIER LIFESTYLE

- Take a baby aspirin to reduce blood clots.
- Maintain a healthy weight.
- Drink no more than one alcoholic drink per day.
- Sleep seven or eight hours each night.
- Don't smoke. It causes one in five deaths in the United States.
- Wear your seat belt. More than half of people who die in car wrecks aren't wearing them.
- While driving, avoid distractions (especially cell phones, children, and eating) to prevent one out of four accidents.
- Stay out of the midday sun and wear sunscreen to reduce skin aging and cancer.

see sidebar next page

BUILDING A HEALTHIER LIFESTYLE

- If you live alone, adopt a dog or cat to relieve depression, lower blood pressure, promote exercise, and improve survival after heart attack.

- Stay positive: Optimistic people live longer, have shorter head colds, and are less likely to get dementia.

look outside. Women need to be aware of the ways the media manipulates them and learn to think for themselves.

If something is bothering her, a woman needs to look honestly at herself — and not just because the media says she's imperfect. Then she needs to do something about it, and have some fun while she's at it. By putting herself in charge of her mind and body makeover she can restructure her thoughts and start taking risks. Implementing a financial plan and improving her relationships may take her out of her comfort zone but she will feel so much more alive, confident, and revived.

· ·

When you think to yourself, 'if only' or 'what if,' I say, 'please don't go there.' Every moment wasted looking back keeps us from moving forward.

Senator Hillary Clinton suspending her presidential campaign,
June 2008

· ·

Life is too short to for a woman to feel bad about herself, so she needs to dump the old messages of the past that keep her from feeling great. By identifying her negative self-statements she can stop them now and replace them with the things she likes about herself: a great smile, great sense of humor, wisdom, skills, hopes, dreams, or the kindness she shows to others. Each woman has the power to change into the person she most wants to be.

Rather than waiting for something else to happen before she creates the life she wants, she can start right now. This minute. Now is the best of all possible times to create a healthy environment that is free of the toxic nouns (the people, places, and things) that make us sick.

By showing the universe what she wants a woman can have it for herself today. Behave with goodness to receive goodness. Send out love to receive love. Become a supportive mentor to find a supportive mentor. Act like a successful, competent, capable woman to become one. The toxic messages from media or society can be ignored and a woman can feel fine about her looks and her age.

The end of this story can mark the beginning of the most wonderful chapter of a woman's life journey. The wonderful and smart women reading this book know it is time to make their dreams come true by starting with one small change. What's it going to be?

Resources

HOW TO START A TIMELESS WOMEN GROUP

1. Select a comfortable environment where participants can speak freely.
2. Invite six to eight women friends or acquaintances; they may be of various ages.
3. Designate a facilitator for each gathering who will make sure everyone has an opportunity to speak.
4. Agree upon start and end times.
5. Select a few topics from the Timeless Women discussion guide before the meeting.
6. At the first meeting, have each person introduce herself and say why she is interested in the topic.
7. Before ending the gathering, have someone summarize the discussion.
8. Agree upon the next gathering time and select a topic.
9. Share email addresses for easy organization.

TIMELESS WOMEN SPEAK DISCUSSION QUESTIONS

- How do you feel about aging now, compared to when you were younger? How often do you think about getting older? What do you think of most often?

- Are you afraid of getting older? Are you afraid of dying? Which scares you more?

- What situations/activities most often cause you to think about getting older?

- What do you do or say to yourself that helps your feelings?

- How did your mother (or other primary female caretaker) feel about getting older? What did she do to manage her feelings?

- How much do your feelings about getting older resemble your mother's feelings about getting older?

- What other role models have you had regarding aging, other than your mother?

- When you think about getting older, what is your greatest concern now?

- Are there fears or worries about aging that you had in the past that you have overcome? What were they? How did you overcome them?

- When you think about getting older, what do you look forward to most?

- What kinds of things are you doing to prepare for successful aging?

- Do you feel your healthcare provider listens carefully to your health concerns?

- In thinking about growing old, what money factors concern you?

- If you work now, at what age do you plan to stop working for pay? What will make it possible for you to stop?

- What aspects of your appearance are concerns as you get older?

- What aspects of your self-image are most important to you as you get older?

- Have you ever felt "invisible" compared to when you were younger? In what circumstances?

- What most often helps you feel good about yourself?

FIND UPDATED RESOURCES AND MORE INFORMATION
ONLINE AT WOMENSPEAK.COM

- Bibliography and suggested reading
- Information about feeling youthful, relationships, finances, and health
- How to take part in the research and detailed results
- Dr. Nancy's speaking schedule
- Location for Timeless Women Radio

We welcome you to become a part of the WomenSpeak project. We want to hear your voice.

Research Results

WOMEN'S FEAR OF GETTING OLDER AND MAJOR AGING CONCERNS

This table combines data from several survey questions. Women were asked to select their major aging concern from an offered list. Only a few selected "maintaining a youthful appearance" as their top issue, and this percentage is reported in the women of all ages data set. However, many more women identified on other survey items that they were concerned about their "appearance," which we took to mean they wanted to look their best at any age. This figure is represented in the age-cohort data sets. Fear of getting older was reported in a separate question.

Of All Ages	Percent
Fear of getting older	45.1
Having health problems	29.4
Not having enough money	26.0
Being alone	10.1
Loss of psychological/emotional well-being	7.8
Not having a mate	7.1
Financial ignorance	2.4
Having a spiritual void	4.7
Fear of dying	4.1
Losing youthful physical appearance	4.1
Society's view of you as an aging citizen	2.8
Other	1.4

Ages 20-29	Percent
Fear of getting older	58.3
Money	28.6
Health	18.9
Psychological well-being	13.0
Family	13.0
Being alone/no mate	10.0
Appearance	9.5
Self	5.0

Ages 30-39	Percent
Fear of getting older	51.2
Health	33.5
Money	26.1
Appearance	17.1
Family	13.2
Being alone/no mate	7.7
Self	6.3
Psychological well-being	4.8

Ages 40-49	Percent
Fear of getting older	42.7
Health	31.4
Money	27.8
Appearance	14.1
Family	9.7
Being alone/no mate	8.7
Self	6.5
Psychological well-being	0

Ages 50-59	Percent
Fear of getting older	46.9
Health	36.7
Money	26.6
Appearance	8.2
Psychological well-being	6.5
Being alone/no mate	5.7
Family	4.4
Self	3.8

Ages 60-69	Percent
Health	40.0
Fear of getting older	24.6
Money	17.8
Self	12.7
Psychological well-being	8.9
Being alone/no mate	6.6
Appearance	1.8
Family	1.8

Ages 70+	Percent
Fear of getting older	22.6
Health	14.3
Being alone/no mate	14.2
Money	9.5
Psychological well-being	9.5
Appearance	3.3
Family	0
Self	0

Index

About the Authors

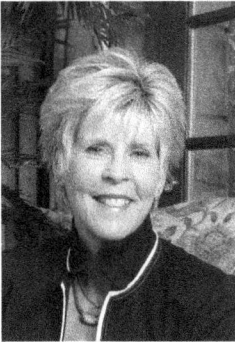

Clinical psychologist Nancy D. O'Reilly, PsyD founded the WomenSpeak Project based on more than 10 years of research. She has worked with women in a strategic, problem-solving fashion for more than 25 years and is passionate about empowering women of all ages to live fearlessly. She hosts the weekly radio show *Timeless Women Speak.*

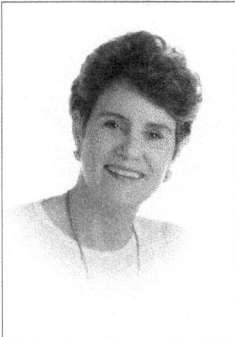

Prize-winning journalist and author Margaret U. Castrey, BA Psychology, has helped tell people's stories and has been active in women's issues for more than 30 years. Editor of the WomenSpeak Project since 2000, she co-authored Dr. O'Reilly's professional journal articles and co-hosts the *Timeless Women Speak* radio show.